MILADY'S AESTHETICIAN SERIES

Aging Skin

MILADY'S AESTHETICIAN SERIES

Aging Skin

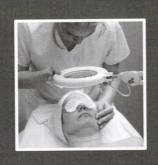
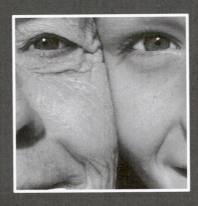
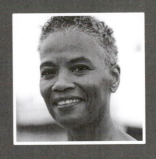

CENGAGE
Learning

SUSANNE SCHMALING, L. E.

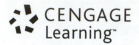

Milady's Aesthetician Series: Aging Skin
Susanne Schmaling, L. E.

President, Milady: Dawn Gerrain

Acquisitions Editor: Martine Edwards

Senior Product Manager: Jessica Mahoney

Editorial Assistant: Elizabeth Edwards

Director of Beauty Industry Relations: Sandra Bruce

Executive Marketing Manager: Gerard McAvey

Content Project Management: PreMediaGlobal

Production Director: Wendy Troeger

Art Director: Benjamin Gleeksman

Compositor: PreMediaGlobal

For product information and technology assistance, contact us at **Professional & Career Group Customer Support, 1-800-648-7450**

For permission to use material from this text or product, submit all requests online at **cengage.com/permissions**.

Further permissions questions can be e-mailed to **permissionrequest@cengage.com**

Library of Congress Control Number: 2011923975

ISBN-13: 978-1-4354-9614-9

ISBN-10: 1-4354-9614-0

Milady

5 Maxwell Drive

Clifton Park, NY 12065-2919

USA

Cengage Learning products are represented in Canada by Nelson Education, Ltd.

For your lifelong learning solutions, visit **milady.cengage.com**

Visit our corporate website at **cengage.com**.

Notice to the Reader

Publisher does not warrant or guarantee any of the products described herein or perform any independent analysis in connection with any of the product information contained herein. Publisher does not assume, and expressly disclaims, any obligation to obtain and include information other than that provided to it by the manufacturer. The reader is expressly warned to consider and adopt all safety precautions that might be indicated by the activities described herein and to avoid all potential hazards. By following the instructions contained herein, the reader willingly assumes all risks in connection with such instructions. The publisher makes no representations or warranties of any kind, including but not limited to, the warranties of fitness for particular purpose or merchantability, nor are any such representations implied with respect to the material set forth herein, and the publisher takes no responsibility with respect to such material. The publisher shall not be liable for any special, consequential, or exemplary damages resulting, in whole or part, from the readers' use of, or reliance upon, this material.

Printed in the United States of America
1 2 3 4 5 6 7 15 14 13 12 11

Dedication

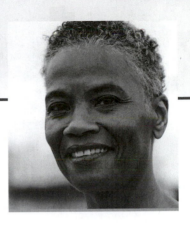

This book is dedicated to all of the amazing estheticians out there. I have met so many beautiful people in this industry that have helped me grow, dream, and believe in myself. I hope I can give just a little bit back.

Contents

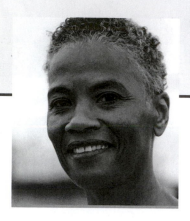

SECTION 3

Chapter 6

■ Chapter 10

■ Chapter 11

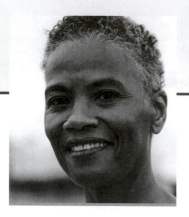

Preface

Writing *Milady's Aesthetician Series: Aging Skin* has been the most challenging project that I have undertaken within my esthetic career. Many people asked what I could possibly add that has not been already written; this is something I thought about quite often. What I found missing is a book with all of the existing information in one place with an esthetic point of view. There are so many different theories on aging, how to prevent it, reverse it, and generally live longer. Trying to find actual non-biased scientific information both in the esthetic realm and the medical realm was very challenging.

Also missing was a practical guide on how to apply this information in a treatment room, spa, salon, and medical spa. The bottom line for every treatment an esthetician performs is the results. How to get those results is often unclear. Working with a clientele that is aging also brings up issues of lifestyle and emotional concerns that estheticians are not trained to handle. The skin is an amazing self-regenerating organ that shows the effects of not only what we eat or how we move, but also what we think. Emotional stress has highly detrimental effects on the health of the skin as well as the body. An esthetician must know how to address these issues with the client.

Many of you may have different ideas about what is considered effective anti-aging therapy. If those modalities are missing from this book, it is only because the therapies have not been validated by an objective source. That does not mean they are not effective, just unsubstantiated for now. The pace of science is moving so quickly that many of the "alternative" treatments of 10 years ago are now considered mainstream and many of our esthetic modalities are being validated by the new scientific approach to skin care.

Throughout this book you will find the latest accepted theories on aging, and how to apply that knowledge when treating clients. Information on lifestyle, nutrition, fitness, and medical treatments are also provided. The goal is to teach the esthetician how to integrate all aspects of what is currently available to improve an aging body. This does not mean that an esthetician needs to be a nutritionist in order to treat aging skin, only that estheticians should understand how important correct nutrition is to the health of the skin. Many medical treatments listed are not within the scope of practice for an esthetician but the knowledge of these treatments is important to provide comprehensive and effective advice to clients.

Most of the answers an esthetician needs are covered in this book, although new techniques and products are arriving all the time in this industry. There is an extensive section on the physiology of the skin, which will help the esthetician ask some *critical thinking* questions when considering whether or not the products or treatments work. This book will help you ask the questions that will set you apart as an expert in esthetics, which in turn provides the support that your clients deserve.

About the Author

Susanne Schmaling

Susanne Schmaling is a Regional Education Manager for Bioelements professional skin care and the Founder and Director of the Pacific Institute of Esthetics located in Northwest Oregon. The Institute offers advanced skin care training for estheticians, teachers, cosmetologists, massage therapists, medical personnel, and business owners. She is also the author of the critically acclaimed *Milady's Aesthetician Series: The Comprehensive Guide to Esthetic Equipment*, copyright 2009, Milady, a part of Cengage Learning.

With a focus on skin science, dynamic measurable anti-aging skin therapies, and holistic skin care techniques, Susanne's expertise and extensive experience make her a popular presenter at conferences and seminars throughout the world. As a licensed esthetician and former creator and owner of an award-winning day spa, her career includes extensive experience in all aspects of esthetics, spa body therapies, makeup, and nail technology, as well as spa consulting and spa design.

Acknowledgements

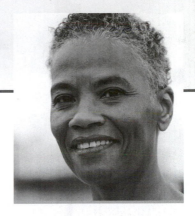

I would like to thank so many people for the help I received writing this book:

Martine Edwards, Acquisitions Editor, Cengage Learning (most awesome woman ever!), Jessica Mahoney, Product Manager, Cengage Learning (book master extraordinaire), the whole editorial team at Milady's, a part of Cengage Learning, MJ Higgins (you know what you did!), Pat Lam (you are a true inspiration to me), Susanne Warfield (industry protector! You need a cape), Rebecca Gadberry (thank you for your knowledge), Barbara Solomone at Bioelements (sharing your limited time and incredible knowledge), Renee Harvey (great esthetician, teacher, and yoga master), and Donna Quinn (wonderful writer, mentor, and friend)

I would like to acknowledge the vendors who gave permission to use their information:

Danielle Tsolkis- Silhouet Tone®

PCA Skin®

Bioelements Professional Skin Care

To my family and friends who put up with me through marathon writing sessions and general neglect, now I will just be a pest!

Jim (I love you, the PCs worked)

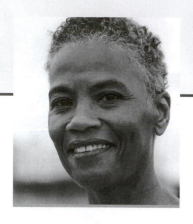

Reviewers

Milady and the author would like thank the following professionals for providing their valuable insight and assistance in the development of the manuscript. This reviewing task is a critical component of the success of a book. We are grateful for your time and honest feedback.

Celia G. Hines, American Spirit Institute, VA

Denise Podbielski, CHHP CHNP, Making Faces, NY

Jean Harrity, Faces By Jean, IL

Jeanne Valek Healy, Medical Esthetician, Instructor, President of Carolina Skin Care Academy, Inc., SC

Judith Culp, CIDESCO Diplomat, NCEA Certified, instructor and CEO of NW Institute of Esthetics, OR

Linda Burmeister, International Dermal Institute/Dermalogica, Inc., CA

Shelley Hess, Holistic Esthetician, Facemaker Enterprises, CA

Tina M. Zillmann, VP and Educational Director for Skin Rejuvenation Clinique Inc. / Advanced Rejuvenating Concepts, TX

Tracy L. Johnson, Tracy Johnson Skin Care Company, GA

Basics of Aging

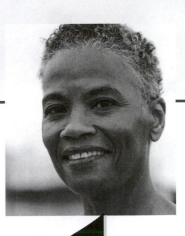

SECTION CONTENTS

Section 1

1

Estheticians and the Holistic Approach to Aging

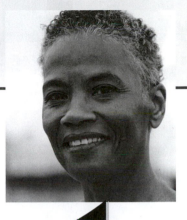

Chapter 1

Key Terms

calcitonin gene-
  related peptide
  (CGRP)
estheticians
  (aestheticians)

holistic esthetics
humectant
Langerhans cells
NICE concept
self-objectification

systemic sensitivity
tactile sensitivity

Learning Objectives

After completing this chapter, you will be able to:

1. Identify the esthetician's role in aging skin care.
2. Understand the esthetician's scope of practice.
3. Understand the role that *beauty obsession* has on clients.
4. Understand the holistic approach to aging.

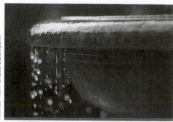

Figure 1–1 Humans have been seeking the fountain of youth for ages.

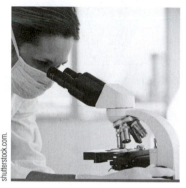

Figure 1–2 Science is making advances in understanding the aging process with the discovery of the DNA code.

esthetician (or aesthetician)
a licensed professional who is an expert on maintaining and improving healthy skin.

■ INTRODUCTION: CAN YOU REVERSE THE SIGNS OF AGING?

Throughout history including the time of Ponce de Leon and the fountain of youth, mankind has looked for a way to reverse and stop the aging process. Currently, we are obsessed with anti-aging medical treatments and staying young (Figure 1–1). Why humans have the need to fight aging has been hotly debated and will continue to be. Experts focus on many reasons including fear of death, loss of both mental and physical control as we age, and loss of sex appeal.

The anti-aging market is a multibillion dollar industry that continues to grow even in the midst of a recession. An entire body of science has been created that focuses solely on how to prevent and reverse the aging process. Just as in times past, many of the ideas and therapies amount to magic or snake oil.

There is an interesting trend in this body of science that may one day prove to be the true fountain of youth. These advances have been made by scientists cracking the DNA code. The more they learn about how we are made, the more they learn about how we age.

At this time there is no way to reverse aging, but we can slow it down. Just in the last century the average lifespan of an American has increased from 45 years in 1900 to 70 in 2009 (Figure 1–2). This is an incredible evolution especially when you take into account the fact that the lifespan of an average male in the 1700s was 35 years. This is an amazing time to be alive.

The Esthetic Professional's Role

What is an esthetician? How many times have you heard that question throughout your career? The professional skin care industry is in the midst of a major change that will ultimately affect how you answer that question. Identifying and defining what an esthetician is, is important in order to determine what role an esthetician will play with an anti-aging treatment. The line between the medical and esthetic worlds is being blurred, with physicians seeing a new revenue center, and technology creating invasive skin-altering treatments. With that in mind let's look at what we currently recognize as a scope of practice defined by state licensing agencies. One of the most common scope of practice definitions is:

Estheticians or **aestheticians** use their hands or mechanical or electrical apparatuses or appliances for cleansing, stimulating, manipulating, exfoliating or applying lotions or creams for the improvement of skin appearance and for the temporary removal of hair, makeup artistry, facial and body wrapping, and facial and body waxing (Figure 1–3).

In addition to scope of practice, there are industry-defined descriptions. For example;

- An esthetician is an expert on maintaining and improving healthy skin.
- An esthetician is a qualified beauty professional who works to enhance the skin by applying special products and massage techniques.

A variety of terms are used to describe the professional. You will see *esthetician* and *aesthetician*, *beauty therapist* and *skin care therapist*. Is there a difference in meaning? Many people do not think so. The dictionary defines *aesthetician* as a specialist in aesthetics. When you look closely at the term aesthetics you find that it directly relates to a branch of philosophy that focuses on the nature of beauty and the appreciation of art, culture, and taste.

There has been a movement within the last 20 years to define a new category for the esthetician that signifies more advanced knowledge and experience. The titles used are *paramedical aesthetician*, *clinical esthetician*, and *medical aesthetician*. Regardless of the titles, the scope of practice remains the same. This statement sums it up best: "an (aesthetician, esthetician, skin therapist, or medical aesthetician) is a licensed professional who is an expert on maintaining and improving healthy skin." The key here is healthy skin. An esthetician will not treat or diagnose any skin disease, or alter the structure and function of the skin without the supervision of a doctor. With that in mind let's look at the role of an esthetician in treating an aging client.

In the skin care clinic, spa, medical spa, and salon anti-aging treatments are the most frequently requested treatments. In order to provide an effective results-oriented treatment, it is important to understand skin physiology, aging theories, cosmetic chemistry, and basic treatment protocols. Understanding the basic science of the skin allows you to scrutinize whatever is presented as the latest aging miracle in an objective manner. It also allows for effective communication with clients in order to minimize disappointment and meet their needs.

Presently the main esthetic therapeutic approach to aging has been to prevent further damage while addressing the signs of aging present at the time of consultation. Reversing aging is impossible but the tools an esthetician uses such as microdermabrasion, peels, certain technologies, and even massage can improve the appearance of the stratum corneum. When these

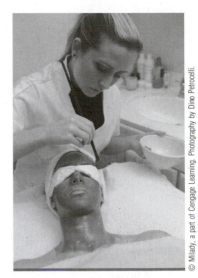

Figure 1–3 An aesthetician/esthetician is a licensed professional who is an expert on maintaining and improving healthy skin.

The spelling of the term esthetician varies based on the type of esthetic services you are performing. Within the medical profession the spelling of *aesthetician* is often used in reference to the Greek word *aesthetikos*, whereas the spelling *esthetician* is used in Western culture to reflect a modern spa culture, and the term beauty therapist is primarily used throughout the world to describe an esthetician.

modalities are stopped, of course, the signs of aging will return. The medical approach is somewhat the same with more intense intervention such as lasers, surgery, and injectables. None of these services can reverse the aging process but they can temporarily correct the appearance of the skin.

The esthetician will be a support through a cosmetic medical process or for some an alternative to the medical approach. There are so many different specialties an esthetician can have that creating a predefined role is not realistic. As long as the esthetician stays within the scope of practice, the client can be appropriately supported. The focus is always on the clients and the healthiest way to support them. We do not want to cause any harm, nor exploit them for financial gain.

▪ THE COST OF BEAUTY OBSESSION

In August 2008 the YWCA, a worldwide multicultural women's organization, published a report called "Beauty at Any Cost" which described the effects of the American culture's obsession with an impossible standard of beauty. This report also detailed the economic impact that such an obsession can make on the finances of women. The report summarized different categories of economic impact such as economic costs, health implications, and interpersonal and personal relationships and detailed the harm that was being done by the pressure to achieve an unrealistic version of beauty. The report is summarized by category.

Economic Costs

Females are spending an incredible amount of money on beauty, money which invested could provide for a substantial retirement. An expectation of physical beauty impacts women economically through *lookism* in their workplaces. Lookism is prejudice based on physical appearance and attractiveness, and is an increasing equal-opportunity problem. This is despite the fact that work productivity has not been scientifically linked with physical attractiveness.[1]

Health Concerns

Health concerns related to the pursuit of beauty include unhealthy dieting, eating disorders, smoking, and drug use. In addition to personal habits, there are risks to health due to medical cosmetic procedures that are often overlooked, such as cardiovascular complications from general anesthesia.

Cosmetic Safety

In the United States, cosmetics are not subject to testing by the U.S. Food and Drug Administration (FDA), and the FDA is not required to give pre-market approval before cosmetics are offered to consumers. Cosmetics companies are not required to register to the FDA information on cosmetics ingredients, or cosmetics-related injuries. Individual cosmetics companies are responsible for substantiating the safety of their ingredients.

Self-esteem

Self-objectification is the tendency for women to judge themselves based on their physical appearance, and they feel that if they do not meet certain physical expectations they will not be accepted by other people. The association between self-objectification and anxiety about appearance and feelings of shame has been found in adolescent girls (12- to 13-year-olds) as well as in adult women. Also, self-objectification has been repeatedly shown to detract from the ability to concentrate and focus one's attention, thus leading to impaired performance on mental activities.[2]

self-objectification
the tendency for women to evaluate themselves based on their physical appearance because they believe that this is how others judge them.

Why Is the *Beauty at Any Cost* Report Important?

Our role as estheticians can put us directly in the position of reinforcing the impossible standards set by our culture not only on our clients but on ourselves. An esthetician can also be put in the position of mitigating the effects of such a standard by not supporting them. Such a stance is not an easy one and requires a good deal of self-esteem. It is also important to understand our clients and the effect this culture has on them. Even though this report seems highly anti-beauty, which can impact the earning potential of an esthetician, by understanding what is happening in this culture we can find a way to work within it in a positive manner.

With any philosophy, the interpretation of information is never black and white. When we look at *aesthetics* as it is defined as a philosophy, we find that the nature of beauty is up for interpretation. The reality is that beauty is in the eye of the beholder. Estheticians are in a perfect position to emphasize the importance of maintaining skin health, which will have the side effect of improving the overall appearance of the client.

We have all experienced that client who only experiences touch when he or she comes in for a facial treatment. Being placed in that

Holistic esthetics
looking at the lifestyle, nutrition, physical fitness and daily care when treating their skin

Humectant
a class of cosmetic ingredients that attract water with in the skin.

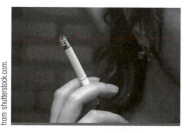

© Zoommer, 2010. Used under license from shutterstock.com.

Figure 1–4 Lifestyle factors must be considered in an aesthetician's holistic approach to anti-aging treatments.

position is a privilege and honor that requires a well-grounded approach to esthetics and interpersonal skills as well.

A question remains that must be pondered by the esthetics community: do we embrace the impossible cultural standards of beauty or do we create a new approach? This does not mean that an esthetician would be anti-beauty and completely discount any treatment, aesthetic medical procedure, or product as damaging. Instead, critical thinking is required when recommending any approach to a client or undergoing treatment ourselves.

The fact remains that we have not yet witnessed a geriatric generation that has undergone this level of invasive aesthetic procedures or anti-aging intervention. The long-term effects of these treatments on an individual's well-being and physical health are relatively unknown. The FDA currently regulates anything that deals with the medical arena with testing for safety, but as we have seen over the years this does not always signify that there are no long-term negative effects.

HOLISTIC APPROACH—AGING GRACEFULLY

What does is mean to age gracefully? Many experts talk about attitude, accepting the inevitable and being flexible with life changes. This is not a bad way to look at it, but for our purposes aging gracefully is a *do what you can without further harm* philosophy. An esthetician's approach is a holistic one. **Holistic esthetics** means looking at the entire person, when treating their skin. The areas that need to be addressed are:

Lifestyle

- Smoking, drinking, daily sun exposure, high stress job, travel schedule, and daily routine (Figure 1–4)
- Working and living environment—high humidity versus climate controlled

Personal Stressors

Medical issues, interpersonal issues, job, and self-esteem (Figure 1–5)

Diet

High fat diet, junk food, supplementation, caffeine, alcohol, and carbonated drinks (Figure 1–6)

Medical History

- Disabilities, physical limitations
- Skin conditions
- Issues such as diabetes, heart disease, autoimmune disease, arthritis, and cancer (Figure 1–7)

Skin Care

- Types of esthetic and medical treatments tried (Figure 1–8)
- Daily habits such as: sleeping in makeup, products used

Activity Level

- Sedentary or consistent exercise, type of exercise (Figure 1–9)

Attitude

- Thoughts on aging
- Life goals (Figure 1–10)
- Expectations of treatment outcome
- Level of commitment to treatment process, self-care

The holistic approach requires an in-depth consultation and extra time, but can make a dramatic difference in the results the client will receive, as illustrated in this example.

If presented with a client who hates to use a daily skin care routine and refuses to exercise or have a healthy diet, yet expects to see a reduction in her symptoms of aging skin by getting monthly facial treatments, you can recommend a better approach that will fit into her current lifestyle and belief system. Meanwhile an esthetician can educate the client on why this will not fully give her the results she seeks without other additional lifestyle modifications. Not only have you avoided having an upset client who has unrealistic expectations, you have also educated her in a way that will build trust and further the long-term client relationship.

Throughout this book you will be gaining knowledge on each part of the holistic esthetic approach. By the end, you will be able to put

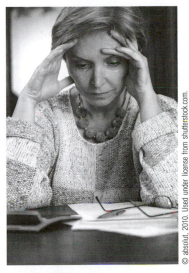

Figure 1–5 Personal stressors affect the well-being of our skin.

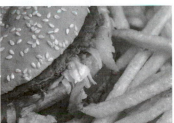

Figure 1–6 Not eating properly also affects the well-being of our skin.

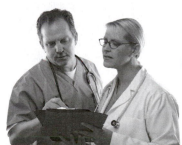

Figure 1–7 Sharing your medical history is important for your treatment.

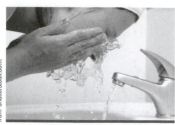

Figure 1–8 Review your current skin care regimen and treatments previously experienced.

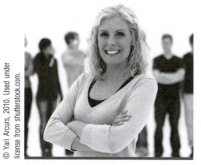

Figure 1–10 The client's attitude about life and self-care can greatly impact the treatment process.

Langerhans cells
important part of the immune system found in skin; digests antigens.

calcitonin gene-related peptide (CGRP)
regulates the antigen presenting function of the Langerhans cells.

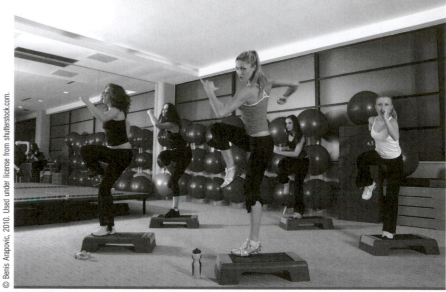

Figure 1–9 Your activity level affects the skin as well.

together your own comprehensive plan for your clients utilizing a team of experts to help you address all areas mentioned.

The Mind–Skin Link

In 1993 Massachusetts General Hospital and Harvard Cutaneous Biology Research Center conducted a study on the possibility of a mind and body connection manifesting symptoms within the skin. This study showed a contact point between **Langerhans cells** in the skin and nerve cells which confirm that the mind and body are connected in the skin. Langerhans cells are an important part of the immune system and known to digest antigens. Langerhans cells contact cutaneous nerves that contain **calcitonin gene-related peptide (CGRP)**, which is a transmitter to regulate the antigen-presenting function of Langerhans cells. This finding showed that Langerhans cells are capable of influencing nerves by producing factors that affect neuron differentiation.[3] This means that a thought of sensitivity sends a message that is translated to the nerves, which in turn activates the Langerhans cells, thus causing the sensitivity reaction.

This was further confirmed by T. Ozawa with the discovery of the existence of a bidirectional regulatory mechanism between the nervous system and the immune system within the skin.[4]

These two studies are just a sample of the many ongoing studies that will further reinforce the esthetician's knowledge of how the mind affects the skin. Estheticians have witnessed the effects of a mind–skin link such as delayed skin barrier repair and irritation. Studies have shown that stress can delay skin barrier function by 20%.[5]

Prolonged anxiety and tension promote secretion of calcitonin gene-related peptide (CGRP) from the pituitary gland, which leads to a reduction of immunological function.

In order to make an improvement in our clients' skin, this mind–skin link needs to be addressed. If the client feels that they are sensitive, they really are.

Some symptoms of stressed skin that may appear are:

- Rough texture resistant to treatment
- Sensitive skin; this can be **tactile sensitivity** or **systemic sensitivity** or both
- Inflammation; both chronic and acute
- Dryness, flakiness, and dehydration (Figure 1–11)
- Feeling of stinging, burning, or general tightness; can occur without inflammation

All of these symptoms can be addressed by understanding the **NICE concept**. The NICE concept states that the nervous, immune, cutaneous, and endocrine systems all work together to activate healthy skin function by the secretion of homeostasin.[6] When one area is impacted, it affects the physiology of the skin in various ways.

Based on this information it is important to address the mind–skin link with clients when creating a healthy aging program. Offer them options for dealing with issues that may affect how they impact their skin and body as well. This can include suggesting the following:

- Meditation (Figure 1–12)
- Biofeedback
- Talk therapy
- Massage
- Art therapy
- Animal-assisted therapy (for example, equine-assisted therapy)
- Spending time in nature

Chapter 2 will give you some further guidelines in dealing with some of the uncomfortable situations that you may face in the treatment room. Aging is a highly emotional process for some people, and learning how to recognize and deal with clients who have these emotions will protect you and your client.

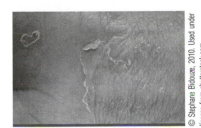

Figure 1–11 Science has identified the connection between the nervous system and the immune system within the skin.

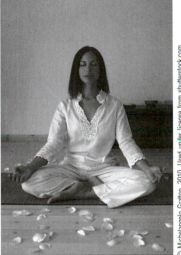

Figure 1–12 Options for reducing stress include meditation, massage, and various forms of therapy.

> Always recommend that the clients see a licensed professional, such as a therapist or psychologist, when concerned about depression, anxiety, and grief issues. An esthetician does not have the training to recognize when a client is in crisis.

tactile sensitivity
client feels uncomfortable when certain fabrics or pressures are used on the skin. Even towels can feel uncomfortable.

systemic sensitivity
Sensitive to environmental insults; internal sensitivity; can be made worse by allergies, medication and disease; sensitivity caused by internal factors.

NICE concept
concept which states that the nervous, immune, cutaneous and endocrine systems all work together to activate healthy skin function by the secretion of homeostasin.

▶ ⟩ ⟩ Top Ten Tips to Take to the Clinic

1. We cannot stop or reverse the aging process, only slow it down.

2. Remember to always work within your state's scope of practice. It is important to understand clients and the effect the beauty culture has on their self-esteem.

3. Cosmetics are not subject to testing by the U.S. Food and Drug Administration (FDA).

4. Holistic esthetics means looking at the entire person, when treating their skin.

5. There is a contact point between Langerhans cells in the skin and nerve cells which confirm that the mind and body are connected in the skin.

6. It is important to address the mind–skin link with a client when creating a healthy aging program.

7. Offer your clients options for dealing with issues that may affect their skin and body health.

8. Understand the NICE concept, which states that the nervous, immune, cutaneous, and endocrine systems all work together to activate healthy skin function by the secretion of homeostasin.

9. Always recommend that the clients see a licensed professional, such as a therapist or psychologist, when concerned about depression, anxiety, and grief issues.

10. If clients feel that they are sensitive, always treat the sensitivity first.

Chapter Review Questions

1. What is one of the definitions of *esthetician*?

2. Can an esthetician diagnose or treat any skin disease?

3. What are the areas of a client's life that need to be considered when approaching aging treatment holistically?

4. Can an esthetician offer advice to clients dealing with depression, anxiety, or grief issues?

5. What are the signs of sensitive skin?

References

1. YWCA USA. (2008). *Beauty at Any Cost: The Consequences of America's Beauty Obsession on Women and Girls.* Retrieved from http://www.ywca.org.
2. YWCA USA. (2008). *Beauty at Any Cost: The Consequences of America's Beauty Obsession on Women and Girls.* Retrieved from http://www.ywca.org.
3. Schueller, R., and Romanowski, P. (2009). *Beginning Cosmetic Chemistry*, 3rd Edition. Carol Stream, IL: Allured Publishing, 471–477.
4. Schueller, R., Romanowski, P. (2009) *Beginning Cosmetic Chemistry*, 3rd Edition. Carol Stream IL: Allured Publishing; pgs 471–477.
5. Schueller, R., Romanowski, P. (2009) *Beginning Cosmetic Chemistry*, 3rd Edition. Carol Stream IL: Allured Publishing; pgs 471–477.
6. Schueller, R., Romanowski, P. (2009) Beginning Cosmetic Chemistry, 3rd Edition. Carol Stream IL: Allured Publishing; pgs 471–477.

Working with a Healthy Aging Client

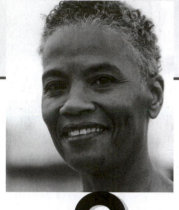

Key Terms

fibromyalgia   mid-life   professionalism
interpersonal skills   astonishment

Learning Objectives

After completing this chapter, you will be able to:

1. Understand the basics of good communication and will listening.
2. Understand why professionalism and ethics are important to skin care professionals.
3. Learn how to work with physically challenged clients.
4. Understand the effects of aging on self-esteem.
5. Learn tips about marketing to healthy aging clients.

▪ INTERPERSONAL SKILLS

Working with clients can be one of the most rewarding and challenging things that an esthetician can experience (Figure 2–1). Learning how to effectively deal with all kinds of people and situations is an often overlooked skill set. Most people who enter this profession have a natural ability to interact with clients and genuinely want to help them; those who do not develop good **interpersonal skills** generally do not last long in this industry. Even if you have a natural ability to interact with people in a positive manner there will be situations that will challenge everything you think you know about people. Having tools to access can make a challenging situation easier to handle.

Positive Communication Skills

Positive communication with your client is as important as being skilled at the technical side of your job. Most challenges arise from miscommunication and unrealistic expectations. It is important to master the basics of good communication. They include:

Listening

Listening is the most important skill to master. It is common to think that clients are listening, but often they miss the core subject of the conversation. Internal issues and biases can interfere with the client's interpretation of a conversation and can lead to client disappointment and frustration. To be an effective listener, there are some key steps to follow:

Ask open-ended questions   Ask the client open-ended questions, such as 'What are your most important skin concerns?" Avoid yes or no questions, for example, "I see that you are concerned with aging issues from your intake form, is that correct?" An open-ended question allows the dialogue to start and the client relationship begins to build trust.

Maintain eye contact and positive body language   Eye contact will help put your clients at ease and make them feel welcome.

Do not interrupt during conversation   This task can be difficult when you have clients who need to vent their feelings, and you have only a short amount of time with them. It is important for clients to feel that they are the focus of your attention, and interrupting the conversation when time is tight can be difficult. This is where reframing or summarizing the conversation will be important.

Keep the focus on the client   Giving information about your experiences in order to show a client you empathize with them takes the focus

interpersonal skills
ability to interact with clients.

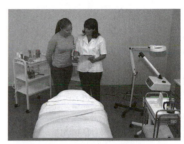

© Milady, a part of Cengage Learning.
Photography by Rob Werfel.

Figure 2–1 Interpersonal skills are a necessary part of successfully managing client communications.

away from them. Try instead to ask questions about their feelings or interpretations of the issue to get a clearer picture of what they need. For example:

> Try saying this: "I understand that you are concerned with your skin. How do you feel about your skin right now?"

> Don't say this: "I understand that you are concerned with the aging of your skin. I woke up this morning with new crow's feet and tried this new cream which helped immediately. You should really try this."

If you try the approach I do not recommend, which turns the focus away from the client, you will miss the opportunity to find out that this client's concern is actually focused on prevention and feeling healthy, and that the client is under a tremendous amount of stress from life style issues. This information would refocus the comprehensive treatment plan to make it more effective.

Clear Verbal Communication

In order to have clear verbal communication with your client, it is important to keep the industry terms and slang to a minimum. Clear, concise language that conveys your message will be most effective. Slang changes with every trend and generation but some examples to avoid include:

> "My bad."
> "Whatever!"
> "What's up?"
> "Roger."
> "Cool."
> "Dig it."

Industry terms are another area of concern. You should not dumb down your communication, as everyone resents being patronized, but you should be aware that the client may have no idea what *gly peel* means or what the *physiology of the skin* is. It is easy to try to give too much information to the client right from the first consultation. This is why listening is so important. You may find out that your client is familiar with the industry and understands more than you think or may be new to getting this type of care. Choose your vocabulary based on the information provided by the client during the consultation.

Communicating with Co-workers   Communicating with fellow co-workers is also an important skill to develop. Many estheticians who are working with an aging clientele are working in a medical setting as well. Many books and seminars are given on how to work within that setting, and much emphasis is put on how an esthetician should communicate with a physician due to their differences in education.

The reality is that doctors, nurses, and others in the medical profession are human beings as well. Even though a licensed esthetician may have fewer years of education than a doctor, this does not imply that the esthetician as a person is less intelligent or unable to communicate with medical personnel. The same communication guidelines that work with a client can be effective with co-workers as well. When speaking to co-workers including a doctor or related medical professionals, keep in mind the following guidelines:

- Be direct. Have a clear goal in mind when approaching someone.
- Be honest. Do not be afraid to give a dissenting view. Do not change the facts to make someone feel better or to avoid an uncomfortable situation.
- Be professional. You are an expert in your field. If you do not understand a situation, admitting that you do not understand does not diminish your reputation, as long as you are learning.
- Respect each individual's time. Lengthy illustrated questions take up too much time and can be confusing.
- Keep personal information to a minimum.
- Do not gossip.
- Use appropriate terminology. Medical terminology is used in a medical setting. Esthetic terminology is used in a spa, salon, or skin-care clinic setting. For example, using the term *couperose* with a doctor will get you an exasperated look, where *telangiectasia* will get a better response. The same concept applies when talking to clients; do they know what *telangiectasia* is?

Positive Body Language

How you use body language is as important as what you say. Everyone has experienced someone conveying one message in words and the opposite in body language. For example, if someone says, "How are you feeling today?" while looking away, their body language shows lack of interest. The meaning is changed when accompanied by different types of body language. Here are a few guidelines for positive body language with your clients:

- Maintain direct eye contact.
- Shake hands or gently touch the client on the shoulder.
- Smile, and speak calmly.
- Face your body towards the client.
- Keep your arms at the sides of your body. Some gesturing during conversation is fine as long as it is not too animated.
- Keep your feet still, and avoid nervous fidgeting.

- Maintain a posture that is correct and relaxed; leaning towards the client is fine as long as personal space is respected.

  This type of body language should be avoided:

- Looking away from client during conversation
- Crossing your arms on your chest
- Nervously fidgeting
- Poor pronunciation and mumbling
- Facing away from client
- Hiding hands when speaking
- Invading a client's personal space

Summarizing or Reframing Communication   The best way to clarify what you are hearing is to summarize what was said back to the client. Sometimes clients can understand that they need to clarify their statements only when you summarize their statements for them. Let's look at an example of a conversation held during an initial consultation:

Esthetician: "Hi Mrs. J, I am _____, your esthetician." (Smile and shake hands.)

Client: "Hi, I am _____ (first name). Nice to meet you."

Esthetician: "I am glad to meet you, too. Have a seat." (Direct your client to a comfortable location. A client can feel lost coming into a new setting. Sit facing the client.) "We are going to perform _____ on you today, and I would like to go over your intake form. What concerns you most about your skin right now?"

Client: "Everything concerns me. I feel like I look old, nothing works that I try, and I do not want to get surgery yet."

Esthetician: "You feel like you look old but do not want surgery and are having a hard time trying to figure out a treatment plan that will work? Is that correct?"

At this point the client will reinforce what you have said or correct it. This allows you to continue the conversation in a way that will get you more detail and help you modify the treatment as needed. You will also notice the emotional state of your client, which can help you add additional touches such as aromatherapy for stress reduction or a warm towel under the neck.

This process of summarizing may be repeated several times throughout the consultation. With some clients, depending on the information they are trying to relay, restating information back to them may be repeatedly necessary.

> Do not address your client by their first name unless they introduce themselves that way.

Table 2–1 Steps to Communicate with Clients

Good Communication	Actions
Active listening	Ask open-ended questions.
	Do not interrupt during conversation.
	Keep the focus on the client.
Clear verbal communication	Use clear, concise language.
	Do not use slang.
	Be direct.
	Do not gossip.
Positive body language	Maintain direct eye contact.
	Face your body towards the client.
	Shake hands or gently touch client on the shoulder.
	Respect a client's personal space.
	Keep arms at side of body or use minimal hand movement.
	Smile.
	Speak calmly.
Summarize or reframe communication	Repeat back to the client answers they gave.
	Summarize your interpretation of the conversation back to the client.

© Junial Enterprises, 2010. Used under license from shutterstock.com.

Table 2–1 outlines an overview of the steps appropriate for enhancing interpersonal skills and effectively communicating with clients by using active listening, clear verbal dialog, positive body language, and summarization.

■ PROFESSIONALISM AND ETHICS

Professionalism relates not only to how you perform your job but also the impression that you present to your client. One of the definitions of professionalism is this: the characteristics of a member of a vocation founded by specialized vocational training. The reality is that there is room for interpretation of what a professional is and how they should act. In order for you to be taken seriously not only by your clients but also by others you work with, you need to present yourself as being knowledgeable, well groomed, friendly, trustworthy, and stable.

professionalism
the characteristics of a member of a vocation that has specialized vocational training.

Each profession has accepted guidelines for professionals. With in the esthetics industry there is a movement for defining a set of professional guidelines. Most esthetics associations have a set of ethics or principles that are guidelines for members.

NCEA Code of Ethics

The NCEA is the National Coalition of Esthetic Associations and is actively involved in the legislative process protecting estheticians' rights. They have launched the first national certification program and are working to raise education standards across the nation. Listed below is their code of ethics adopted by the many association members throughout the United States.

Associated Skincare Professionals Code of Ethics

Associated Skincare Professionals is an organization that provides much needed liability insurance for their membership. They are affiliated with the Associated Bodywork and Massage Professionals (ABMP) organization and are an example of one of the many associations within the esthetic industry. Their code of ethics is listed here. You will notice many common industry statements.

These are two examples of codes of ethics used within the esthetic industry. It is important to familiarize yourself with the expectations and provide the information to the client as well. Clients will respond favorably when presented with an esthetician's code of ethics, which can help build a loyal clientele.

An Example of Professional Ethics for Esthetics, by the NCEA or National Coalition of Esthetic Associations

---

CLIENT RELATIONSHIPS

Estheticians* will serve the best interests of their clients at all times and will provide the highest quality service possible.

Estheticians will maintain client confidentiality, keep treatment and documentation records, and provide clear, honest communication.

Estheticians will provide clients with clear and realistic goals and outcomes and will not make false claims regarding the potential benefits of the techniques rendered or products recommended.

Estheticians will adhere to the scope of practice of their profession and refer clients to the appropriate qualified health practitioner when indicated.

SCOPE OF PRACTICE

Estheticians will offer services only within the scope of practice as defined by the state within which they operate, if required, and in adherence with appropriate federal laws and regulations.

Estheticians will not utilize any technique/procedure for which they have not had adequate training and shall represent their education, training, qualifications and abilities honestly.

Estheticians will strictly adhere to all usage instructions and guidelines provided by product and equipment manufacturers provided those guidelines and instructions are within the scope of practice as defined by the state, if required.

Estheticians will follow, at minimum, infection control practices as defined by their state regulatory agency, Centers for Disease Control & Prevention (CDC) and Occupational Safety & Health Administration (OSHA).

PROFESSIONALISM

Estheticians will commit themselves to ongoing education and to provide clients and the public with the most accurate information possible.

Estheticians will dress in attire consistent with professional practice and adhere to the Code of Conduct of their governing board.

*For the purpose of the NCEA Code of Ethics, the use of the term Esthetician applies to all licensed skin care professionals as defined by their state law.

An Example of Professional Ethics for Esthetics, by the Associated Skincare Professionals

CLIENT RELATIONSHIPS

I shall endeavor to serve the best interests of my clients at all times and to provide the highest quality service possible.

I shall maintain clear and honest communications with my clients and shall keep client communications confidential.

I shall acknowledge the limitations of my skills and, when necessary, refer clients to the appropriate qualified healthcare professional.

PROFESSIONALISM

I shall maintain the highest standards of professional conduct, providing services in an ethical and professional manner in relation to my clientele, business associates, healthcare professionals, and the general public.

I shall respect the rights of all ethical practitioners and will cooperate with all healthcare professionals in a friendly and professional manner.

I shall refrain from the use of any mind-altering drugs, alcohol, or intoxicants prior to or during professional sessions.

I shall always dress in a professional manner, proper dress being defined as attire suitable and consistent with accepted business and professional practice.

SCOPE OF PRACTICE

I shall provide services within the scope of practice of my profession as defined by the state within which I practice, and in accordance with applicable federal laws and regulations. I will not employ skin care techniques for which I have not had adequate training and shall represent my education, training, qualifications, and abilities honestly.

I shall be conscious of the intent of the services that I am providing, and shall be aware of and practice good judgment regarding the application of skin care treatments utilized.

I shall be thoroughly educated and understand the physiological effects of the specific skin care techniques utilized in order to determine whether such application is contraindicated and/or to determine the most beneficial techniques to apply to a given individual. I shall not apply skin care techniques in those cases where they may be contraindicated without a written referral from the client's primary care provider.

IMAGE/ADVERTISING CLAIMS

I shall strive to project a professional image for myself, my business or place of employment, and the profession in general.

I shall actively participate in educating the public regarding the actual benefits of skin care.

I shall practice honesty in advertising, promote my services ethically and in good taste, and practice and/or advertise only those techniques for which I have received adequate training and/or certification. I shall not make false claims regarding the potential benefits of the techniques rendered.

Working with Physically Challenged Clients

When working with an aging clientele, physical challenges are bound to be present. This is not limited to obvious disabilities such as paralysis, but also to mobility issues. Limitations in mobility can be present not only with the elderly but can also start to show signs with patients in their 20s. Here are some examples of common physical challenges clients may face and guidelines for an effective treatment.

Arthritis

Osteoarthritis usually starts later in life but a client can start manifesting symptoms in their late 30s. Rheumatoid arthritis can show up in younger clientele. Both are autoimmune conditions, and the effects on the body are pain in joints, and a reduction in mobility especially in the hands. These clients experience constant chronic pain in varying degrees.

Service Tips

Use an electric or hydraulic treatment table, as it can be difficult for the client to climb onto a stationary treatment table, and a stool can make a client feel unsafe. See Figure 2–2 for an example of an electric treatment table.

> Clients with cancer is another physical challenge that estheticians will encounter. Additional training is recommended when working with these clients as they experience side effects from their treatment. Oncology esthetics is a specialty that can be very rewarding.

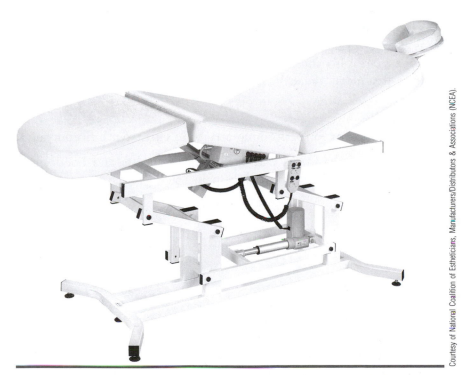

Courtesy of National Coalition of Estheticians, Manufacturers/Distributors & Associations (NCEA).

Figure 2–2 An electric or hydraulic bed eases access on and off the bed.

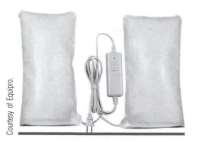

Figure 2–3 A heated pad or mitts provide comfort to many clients.

fibromyalgia
a condition that is defined by widespread muscle pain, fatigue, headaches, sleep disturbance, physiological stress, and problems with thinking.

Use a heated pad and heated mitts during treatment, as heat can naturally lessen the pain if your client is not heat intolerant (Figure 2–3). Menopausal women who are experiencing hot flashes can feel very uncomfortable when heat is applied. Always ask about their comfort level with temperature.

Use a back, neck, and or shoulder support. Depending on their level of disability, clients can experience additional pain when lying completely flat. There are a wide variety of massage bolsters and beds that will adjust to your client. See Figure 2–4 for an example of body support.

Keep home care simple; many clients with arthritis have problems with spreading products on their skin and opening jars. Pumps, sprays, and large wide jars are better for people with severe arthritis. Makeup brush handles should be longer than usual and have a larger handle. Figure 2–5 demonstrates an example of a suitable makeup brush.

Fibromyalgia

According to the Center for Disease Control (CDC) this condition affects approximately 5 million people, the majority being women. **Fibromyalgia** is a condition that is defined by widespread muscle pain, fatigue, headaches, sleep disturbance, physiological stress, and problems with thinking. The pain can be debilitating and when a flare starts, it is often accompanied by extremely sensitive skin, and some clients cannot stand anyone touching their skin. Tingling and numbness are also included in this syndrome. Estheticians seldom perform treatments to clients during a period of full flare.

Service Tips

Here are some tips for performing service to clients with fibromyalgia:

- Use a heated mattress pad and/or heated mitts and booties; the heat can be soothing and reduce pain.

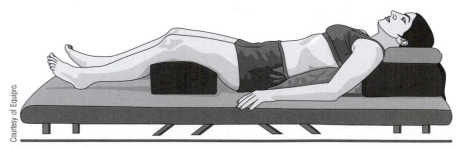

Figure 2–4 Body supports help the client feel more comfortable than laying flat on the bed.

- Use a hydraulic or electric treatment table for easier access.
- Use neck support by offering either a small neck rest or neck support that will cradle the head. The neck support can be removed in the massage phase of the treatment. Headaches are common with fibromyalgia, and supporting the neck can release the muscle spasms that develop.
- Use a light to medium massage strength and focus on the neck, shoulders, and head. Always check with the client about pressure and comfort level. Remember that these clients can be highly sensitive.
- Focus on stress reduction. Use soothing music and low light, because fibromyalgia clients can be environmentally sensitive, especially before a flare. Communicate with your clients about how they are feeling and what your environment is like for them. Even some scents can cause a headache or irritation.

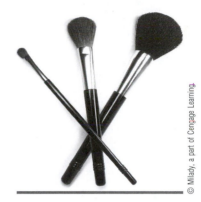

Figure 2–5 Long-handled brushes are easier for ailing hands to use.

Injuries

Anyone can suffer from the ill effects of an injury. Aging clients have a higher number of these effects due to the aging process, and many can experience chronic mobility issues. It is important to always communicate with the client to make sure they are feeling comfortable and not in pain.

Service Tips

Use bolsters under the areas of injury and make sure the client is supported at all times. If there is a shoulder injury, do not forget to support the hands and arms as well.

Use a heated pad, mitts, and/or booties depending on a client's preference and comfort. Be sure to check with the client before applying heat. In some cases it can cause too much inflammation; in others it can be very soothing.

Use a hydraulic or electric treatment table for easy mobility. If you do not have access to a treatment table, have a steady step up, and always support the client getting on and off the treatment table.

Check with the client before massaging an injured area, especially if they have had a head, neck, or upper back injury.

These are just a few of the challenges that a client may present. You will notice that there is some overlap in suggestions. Here is a simple summary to keep in mind regardless of what type of physical challenge your client may be experiencing:

1. Always communicate with your client about how they feel: Is the temperature OK? Are they comfortable? Is the music too loud? Is the lighting too harsh? Ask these questions at the beginning of the service so the

Always support your client with physical challenges on and off the bed. Use a step if you do not have a hydraulic or electric treatment table. Try to invest in a hydraulic or electric treatment table, because the investment will be worth it by making it easier for your clients and saving your back.

client is not interrupted throughout the service. Look for the following body language: fidgeting, raising legs, shallow respiration, flinching when touched in certain areas, and adjusting neck position.

2. Help your client on and off the treatment table.

3. Use heated mattress pads for additional comfort. Just remember to ask your clients how they feel about additional heat. Remember, some menopausal women are going through hot flashes.

4. Keep artificial fragrance to a minimum. Essential oils are fine in moderation. Certain fragrances or overpowering scents can be irritating to people.

5. Use clear written instructions for clients' home care and treatment descriptions. Long, complicated instructions written in small fonts are problematic for clients with failing eyesight, middle-aged eyes, or those under stress. Try to use a 12-point or higher font for easy reading.

6. Keep clutter to a minimum. A clean, well-appointed room will soothe a stressed client and anyone with a physical challenge or with a chronic level of stress.

These simple guidelines will help you provide a comfortable environment for your client. If your clients feel uncomfortable in any way, chances of them rebooking will be slim. This is as important as providing an effective treatment.

THE EFFECTS OF AGING ON SELF-ESTEEM

Self-esteem is an emotional issue at any age, and for some aging can cause a distressing emotional response. For the esthetician, understanding how this affects your client is important not only so you can help them but also so that you can help yourself. Because we all age, we need to know to handle it and how it defines our lives.

Mid-life astonishment (Pearlman, 1993) is one theory that defines what happens to women in late mid-life, usually in their 50s and 60s. This is characterized by an amazement and despair at losing one's physical and sexual attractiveness, multiple losses accompanied by age, awareness of accelerated aging both physically and mentally, and recognizing our culture's stigmatization of aging. This process can lead to a loss of self-esteem, shame, depression, and social isolation (Figure 2–6).[1]

If your client is really invested in appearances, the aging process can be devastating. If your client does not care about appearance, the

mid-life astonishment
theory that defines what happens to women in late mid-life, usually 50s and 60s. This is characterized by an amazement and despair of losing one's physical and sexual attractiveness, multiple losses accompanied by age, awareness of accelerated aging both physically and mentally as well as culture's stigmatization of aging.

aging process could be beneficial as the client grows in maturity and wisdom. In our culture there's a great deal of emphasis on youthfulness and appearances as is described in Chapter 1. Some women seek out a clinician's office for therapy as they are undergoing multiple life changes that make the body changes even more profound. They are experiencing loss of appearance, loss of physical functioning, and loss of social support. Other losses can include financial problems and even spouse and family.

Clients often describe appearance changes caused by aging this way: "I woke up one day and all of a sudden I looked old." They come to the esthetician to try to change this before trying something more invasive. For some, the thought of *getting work done* or *going under the knife* is uncomfortable and vain. They feel some guilt when starting to focus on themselves and are unsure about *what's normal* for an aging face. For example, unwanted hair growth happens to all women but most clients feel that they are afflicted worse than others. The esthetician can at this stage reinforce how normal it is and offer information about the options, which can reduce anxiety.

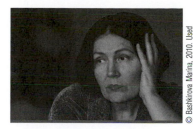

Figure 2–6 Bolsters help protect injuries and areas of pain.

How to Handle Emotions in the Treatment Room

Knowing that aging is an emotional issue for most women is important to understanding how to handle emotional issues in the treatment room. Most estheticians who have been working with clients for years will have stories of emotional breakdowns on the treatment bed or the disclosure of uncomfortable information. Estheticians are not therapists but are often put in the position of therapists. Here are some guidelines from Lana Davis, LCSW, a licensed therapist and social worker who specializes in self-esteem and grief issues. She also recommends spa treatments as part of her client's therapy.

Guidelines for Working with Emotional Clients

- Stay calm.
- Don't try to solve the client's problem.
- Use good listening skills and offer support when appropriate. Often offering a facial tissue and a listening ear will do the trick.
- Do not give advice; stay neutral. For example, say, "I am sorry you are feeling so down, angry, sad, and disappointed." Most of the time, all that is needed is a soothing environment. If the environment is subdued, calm, and relaxing, most of the time all that is needed are simple environmental cues, such as music, tea, water, soothing and comforting items.

- Do not try to be a therapist. Instead, refer your clients to local therapists.
- Limit the conversation. The best thing you can do is say little and give an excellent massage and direct them to breathing and relaxing while you give them their treatment.

Working with a healthy aging clientele is an honor and privilege which requires empathy and understanding as well as technical expertise in esthetics. These guidelines, along with the experience and help of other experienced estheticians, will help an esthetician succeed with their healthy aging clientele.

Marketing to a Healthy Aging Clientele

There are many resources available to help you learn how to market your practice, and estheticians interested in working for themselves should seek out this information. The healthy aging market, which includes the baby boomers, is one of the most profitable. The healthy aging market also requires additional considerations, and here are some tips to help an esthetician to formulate a marketing plan.

Create more than a simple service: these clients need to have their unique concerns and challenges addressed as well their expectations met. Some challenges an aging client may have are as follows:

- ☐ Unrealistic vision of how the client wants to look
- ☐ Poor self-esteem
- ☐ Fear of aging
- ☐ Poor mobility due to arthritis, fibromyalgia, or injuries
- ☐ Poor eyesight
- ☐ Finding skin type–appropriate makeup
- ☐ Getting accurate, unbiased information
- ☐ Not knowing how to correctly take care of his or her skin
- ☐ Finding a professional who understands issues and has technical knowledge

These are just a few of the issues that an esthetician may deal with when marketing to this clientele. In order to be successful it is important to utilize the following marketing principles:

Educate your client. The mature client wants to know why and how. You cannot expect to make a claim of improvement within the skin without explaining the facts.

Listen. Everyone needs to feel that his or her needs are being met. An aging client is also dealing with multiple challenges, which require the esthetician to listen carefully to what the client is trying to express.

Understand. Recognize client challenges and offer solutions. This is the key to offering results-oriented treatments.

Create a service brand. This principle starts with respect, which turns to loyalty that leads to a positive professional–client relationship. Respect from the customer towards you as a professional and from the professional to the client are important. In order to receive respect, key categories of the business must be addressed:

- **Service performance**
  Do you offer quality services and products? Professional skin care products and technology provide an important benefit.
- **Value for the price**
  Including microtreatments or add-ons during a facial treatment for no extra charge is an example. Note: this does not mean that you sacrifice profit.
- **Provide visible results**
  The client needs to see the results of your treatment within the timeline that was advertised to them.
- **Innovation**
  Are you innovative? Additional education is a requirement to build skills that can increase innovation.
- **Reputation**
  Are you respected in your community? How you conduct yourself outside working hours is as important as during them. What pictures and posts do you have on your Facebook page or other social networking websites?
- **Community service**
  Do you give back and get involved? Supporting causes important to the community is valuable for your reputation. Public relations is helpful, in addition to speaking at community groups and schools.
- **Expertise**
  Are you known as an expert in your field?
- **Customer satisfaction**
  Are clients happy with their experience at your business? There will always be an unhappy client, but watch feedback and search the Internet for reviews. Clients may not be telling you how they feel but they will tell everyone they know. Are you making impossible claims about service and products? If you claim *immediate firming* in the skin, be sure you can provide it. Hold manufacturers accountable if they are promising results without proof.
- **Honesty**
  Do you promise more than can be provided? It is best to under-promise benefits and over-deliver results.

- **Reliability**
  Are you reliable to your clients? Showing up on time, ending sessions consistently on time are all-important to the integrity of your business. Do you fulfill commitments made to your clients? If you make a promise, be sure to follow through. For example, if you are going to research questions for a client, get back to the client in a timely manner.
- **Environment**
  Do you offer a secure environment? Clients should feel that their personal information is kept safe and personal conversations will not be shared.

These are all areas to look at when creating a marketing plan for the aging client.

▶ ▷ ▷ Top Ten Tips to Take to the Clinic

1. Practicing positive communication and listening skills prevents miscommunication and unrealistic expectations between you and your client.

2. Develop client relationships and trust by asking open-ended questions and keeping the focus on the client to learn about his or her needs.

3. Use clear, concise language, and avoid slang when consulting with a client.

4. Hold yourself to a high standard of professionalism.

5. Repeat back a summary of what the client has said during the consultation to verify the client's expectations and treatment goals.

6. Understand the common physical challenges clients face and guidelines for an effective treatment.

7. Use a hydraulic or electric treatment table or a step for easier access for clients who are physically challenged or have mobility issues.

8. Always check in with clients to make sure they are comfortable and not experiencing any pain.

9. Maintain a clean, clutter-free room to ensure a comfortable environment for every client.

10. Handle emotional issues in the treatment room when working with a healthy aging clientele by being attentive and remaining neutral and calm.

Chapter Review Questions

1. What are a few basic tips for encouraging positive communication?

2. List ways in which you can portray professionalism and ethics as a skin care professional.

3. Explain ways to accommodate and work with physically challenged clients in the treatment room.

4. What are some of the guidelines for handling emotions in the treatment room?

5. What are some tips for marketing to the healthy aging client?

References

1. Davis, N., Pearlman, S., et al. (1993). *Late Mid-life Astonishment: Faces of Women and Aging*. Binghamton, NY: Haworth Press.

Bibliography

Dietz, B. E. (1996). "The Relationship of Aging to Self-esteem: The Relative Effects of Maturation and Role Accumulation." *International Journal Aging Human Development*: 43 (3): 249–66.

Mizzoni, J. (2010). *Ethics: the Basics*. West Sussex, UK: Wiley-Blackwell.

Rodin, J., and Langer, E. (1980). "Aging Labels: The Decline of Control and the Fall of Self-esteem." *Journal of Social Issues*: 36 (2): 12–29.

Websites

http://www.lovemarks.com
http://www.bbhq.com [search for Boomer Stats]
www.ascpskincare.com
www.ncea.tv

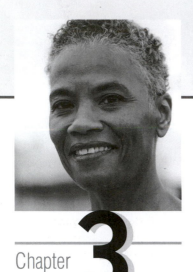

Creating a Healthy Aging Plan

Chapter 3

Key Terms

alipidic
cosmetic sensitivity
desquamation
diffuse redness
elastosis
environmental
    sensitivity
erythema
essential fatty acid
    (EFA)
Fitzpatrick
    classification
folliculitis

Glogau classification
Health Insurance
    Portability and
    Accountability
    Act (HIPAA)
hyperhydrosis
hyperkeratosis
melasma
milia
rhytids
rosacea
Rubin classification
scarred ostia

sebaceous
    hyperplasia
sebaceous secretions
seborrhea
SOAP (Subjective,
    Objective,
    Assessment, and
    Plan)
solar lentigines
tactile sensitivity
telangiectasia

Learning Objectives

After completing this chapter, you will be able to:

1. Perform a healthy aging consultation.
2. Complete a correct skin assessment.
3. Handle and prevent liability issues.

INTRODUCTION

Creating a comprehensive plan for your healthy aging client starts with a correct skin assessment. Without an accurate idea of the state of their skin you will not be able to treat them effectively. This can lead to liability issues due to use of incorrect products and treatments. In this chapter, we will explore how to complete a correct skin assessment as well as what to do if the client experiences a problem during or after a treatment.

CORRECT SKIN ASSESSMENT

Correct skin assessment is an important part of the esthetic treatment, especially when treating aging skin. If a client is given a wrong skin assessment, the entire treatment is compromised. There are so many different systems for skin assessment, and many are based on manufacturer products. This is fine for most clients but can be confusing for estheticians. Most clients have never had an in-depth skin care assessment and are misinformed on the type of skin that they have. This can lead to improper product use and further complicate conditions that the client may have.

In esthetic school most professionals are taught the four basic skin types, related to **sebaceous secretions**. Now a fifth type, sensitive skin, has been added. This is not always accurate but simplifies the assessment process to correlate with products and treatments currently available on the American skin care market. This system is also widely used in the licensing process.

Estheticians also must have knowledge of **Fitzpatrick**, **Rubin**, and **Glogau** classifications, especially when working with physicians. The medical field approaches skin typing in a different manner, by focusing on the visual symptoms of skin disorders—you can see where the esthetician can be confused. These skin typing classifications will be discussed in more detail later in this chapter.

With the changes in aesthetic medicine and cosmetic science creating treatments and products that can cause undesirable side effects, it is time to look at a comprehensive skin assessment program that will be easy to use but take into account a client's healing response as well as genetic skin type. Here is a relatively simple system that will incorporate both the esthetic typing and the medical typing that the esthetician must become familiar with.

This is the first step in determining the process of treatment for an aging clientele. Chapter 5 will explain in detail the treatment options available.

sebaceous secretions
Sebum produced from the sebaceous gland.

Fitzpatrick typing
a skin typing program based on the client's melanin production within the skin. This program can determine a client's ability to heal after aggressive treatments such as chemical peels and lasers.

Rubin classification of aging
aging skin analysis developed by Dr. Mark Rubin.

Glogau Photodamage Classification Scale
developed by Richard G. Glogau, MD, a clinical professor of dermatology at the University of California, San Francisco. It was created in order to objectively measure the severity of photoaging.

Step 1: Determine Skin Type

Identifying the skin type is important for many reasons. Without understanding how much sebaceous activity the skin has, an esthetician is likely to use a product that will not give an optimal outcome. One example is using an emollient anti-aging product on oily skin. During this first step, you will use the magnifying lamp, Woods lamp, or more advanced skin analysis equipment, such as moisture checkers or computer imaging.

There are four types of skin, as outlined in the sections that follow.

Normal Skin

This is a rare skin type and more common in young clients.
Look and touch:

- This type is a skin that is in perfect balance.
- Pores are not large. There will be normal sebaceous secretions seen under a Woods lamp. The key is balanced.
- Texture is smooth, and the skin has a good tone.
- There will be no conditions associated with this skin type.
- Under a Woods lamp, the skin will show an even blue fluorescence.

Ask:

- After cleansing, ask the client, Does your skin feel tight or dry? The answer should be no.

Dry Skin

alipidic
oil dry skin.

Another term for dry is **alipidic**. This refers to skin that has little or no sebaceous secretions.
Look and touch:

- Pores are fine, almost invisible.
- Texture is smooth and fine.
- Under a Woods lamp, the skin will show a white fluorescence

Ask:

- After cleansing, ask the client: Does your face feel uncomfortable? The answer should be yes.
- Do you find that a very emollient cream absorbs quickly? The answer should be yes.
- Do you feel as if you can never get enough moisture? Generally, the answer should be yes.

Combination Skin

This is the most common type. This skin will have additional conditions that will determine which machine and products to use.

Look and touch:

- Pore size can range from small to large, but are located only through the center panel of the face, the typical T-zone.
- Texture can be rough in some areas and smooth in others.
- There will be conditions associated with this skin type.
- Under a Woods lamp the skin will show small orange dots where sebum is being produced. You will also see areas of white fluorescence, which indicates the dry areas.

Ask:

- Do you generally feel tight and dry in some areas and oily in other areas of the face?

Oily Skin

This skin type usually has many conditions associated with it.

Look and touch:

- Pore size is large and visible throughout the face.
- Texture can feel like an orange peel, rough and thick.
- Tone will have a shine with obvious oil.
- There are no areas of dryness, but can be dehydrated.
- Under a Woods lamp you will see small orange dots throughout the face.

Ask:

- Do you feel that you need to wash your face during the day?

Step 2: Determine Fitzpatrick Skin Type or Healing Response Time

Fitzpatrick skin types are used to determine a client's potential reaction to an advanced clinical treatment by estimating a client's genetic background and reaction to UV exposure. This is a useful tool to determine a client's tolerance and potential reaction to a facial treatment, especially skin resurfacing. It is also a guideline to recognizing a more sensitive skin, healing ability, and keloid scarring. Manufacturers also use this typing system when developing laser, IPL machines, and some LED machines. They calibrate programs in the machine to each different skin type. See Figures 3–1 and 3–2 for the Fitzpatrick skin type chart and skin type examples.

Skin Type	UV Exposure	Characteristics	Possible Reactions
Skin Type I	Always burns, never tans; usually burns within 10–15 minutes	White, very fair, red or blond hair, blue eyes, freckles likely	Sensitivity to topical products, the environment, heat, cold, and wind
Skin Type II	Burns easily, tans minimally; usually burns within 30–40 minutes	Fair-skinned, blue, green, or hazel eyes, blond, dishwater blond, or red hair	Rarely develop post-inflammatory pigmentation, least defense against UV damage
Skin Type III	Sometimes burns, gradually tans; usually burns within 60–70 minutes	Cream-white, fair with any eye or hair color, very common coloring	
Skin Type IV	Rarely burns, gradually tans	Brown skin, brown eyes, Mediterranean, southern European, Hispanic	More susceptible to pigmentation problems and keloid scarring, greater defense against environmental & UV damage
Skin Type V	Tans	Dark brown skin, brown-black hair, brown eyes, Asian, Indian, some Africans	
Skin Type VI	Tans well	Black skin, black hair, brown-black eyes, Africans	

Figure 3–1 Fitzpatrick skin types and possible reactions.

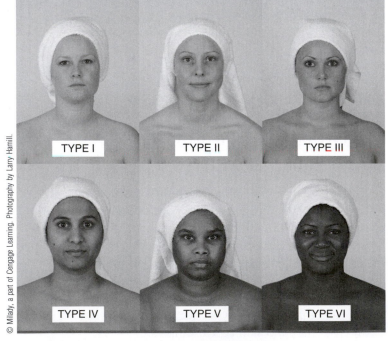

Figure 3–2 Photo examples of Fitzpatrick skin types.

© Milady, a part of Cengage Learning.

© Milady, a part of Cengage Learning. Photography by Larry Hamill.

Another option that is gaining attention is determining the client's healing response time. This is in response to the fact that our genetic background is becoming more and more diverse, and categorizing clients based on skin pigmentation does not always accurately predict the healing response time. To determine a client's healing response some questions to ask are the following:

- Do you bruise easily?
- How long does it take to heal from a cut?
- Do discolorations form after the cut heals?
- Do discolorations form after having a blemish?
- Have you had **melasma** from pregnancy?
- Do you scar easily?
- Is it keloid scarring or atrophic scarring?
- Have you had aesthetic medical treatments such as lasers, IPL, radiofrequency, or plastic surgery?
- How did your skin react after the treatment?

If your client answers *yes* to any of the questions or has had past negative reactions to aesthetic medical treatments, treat the client as a darker Fitzpatrick type regardless of the skin color. This means that invasive or aggressive treatments should be avoided or modified to limit the possible damage.

Step 3: Determine Skin Conditions

Conditions are disorders of the skin and generally what will send a client to seek professional help. Most of the treatments that we use are focused on correction of the skin. In this list is terminology that we use in esthetics mixed with medical terminology. Estheticians work in both fields, so it is important to learn how to clinically document conditions as well as translate to the client. Some of the conditions listed are not considered conditions by the medical community; but are conditions estheticians primarily treat. Use your magnifying loupe as well as the Woods lamp or other advanced skin analysis equipment to look at several areas.

Vascular Conditions

These conditions are related to the microcirculation within the skin. They appear as redness and inflammation in various areas. Clients will visibly notice this and comment on it. The conditions include the following:

- **Telangiectasia** (couperose, broken capillaries)
- **Diffuse redness** (this can indicate a sensitive skin)

melasma
pregnancy mask.

telengiectasia
couperose, or broken capillaries.

diffuse redness
also known as *erythema*, general redness in the skin. This can indicate a sensitive skin.

As our population grows and merges, genetic skin typing is becoming difficult or more difficult may be better here. It is more important to determine a client's reaction to UV sun exposure. Even if they do not tan or have current exposure, ask about childhood UV exposure and current reactions to any chemical or manual peels, cosmetic treatments, and environmental irritants that they may have had.

> Rosacea is a medical disorder that requires the attention of a dermatologist. Do not work outside the esthetic scope of practice and try to treat this disorder.

> Acne grades III and IV should be treated by a dermatologist.

erythema
Also known as *diffuse redness*; increased circulation within the skin that manifests as redness.

rosaceaa
chronic skin condition inflammation of nose cheeks, chin and forehead.

essential fatty acid
Fatty acids found to be essential for proper cellular functions. These are often identified as omega acids 3 and 6, found in fatty fish, some nuts and oils.

seborrhea
an inflammatory skin disorder affecting the scalp, face, and trunk causing scaly, flaky, itchy, red skin.

folliculitis
ingrown hair.

milia
term for whiteheads.

scarred ostia
scarred follicles.

sebaceous hyperplasia
a disorder of the sebaceous glands in which they become enlarged causing clogged pores and raised milia-like bumps.

solar lentigines
freckles.

- **Erythema**
- **Rosacea** (Stage I, II, III)

Lipid System Conditions

These conditions are related to the amount of sebum secretions within the skin. Every skin you see may have some of these common conditions. Clients are particularly sensitive to these conditions due to the impact on their appearance and want them corrected quickly.

- Comedones (open and closed)
- Acne (papules and pustules) grades I, II, III, IV
- **Essential fatty acid (EFA)** deficiency
- **Seborrhea**
- **Folliculitis** (ingrown hair)
- **Milia** (whiteheads), cysts
- **Scarred ostia** (scarred follicles)
- **Sebaceous hyperplasia**

Pigmentation Conditions

These conditions are related to the production of melanin in the skin. They can be caused by UV damage or influenced by hormones. Pigmentation conditions are challenging to treat and are generally accompanied by other aging conditions.

- Hyperpigmentation
- Hypopigmentation
- **Solar lentigines** (freckles)
- Melasma (pregnancy mask)
- Post-inflammatory pigmentation

Aging Conditions

Many advanced treatments are targeted to correct these conditions. It is also the largest group in the population at this time and the focus of this book. The simplest system to use is the Rubin system, which will give you general guidelines on assessing photodamage. Chapter 5 will go into detail about the conditions seen in aging skin and treatment options available.

- Rubin classification system (Table 3–1)
- Glogau classification of aging—this system is used to assess photodamage within the skin, but is complicated and not effective for esthetic treatment (Table 3–2)

Table 3–1 The Rubin system gives general guidelines for assessing photodamage.

Level	Characteristics	Explanations
One–minor aging	Pigmentation and rough, dull texture, thicker stratum corneum, few if any wrinkles	Minor sun damage
Two–moderate aging	Irregular skin color, thick skin, pigmentation changes, actinic keratosis	Wrinkles found around eyes, nasolabial folds deepen, crinkling of skin, loss of elasticity
Three–severe aging	Thick leathery appearance, yellow tint and pebbly texture, open comedones	Wrinkled at rest, loss of elasticity

Table 3–2 The Glogau scale evaluates the photodamage to the skin based on wrinkling.

Glogau Classifications of Photodamage

Type I	Type III
No wrinkles while client is at rest or while moving	Wrinkles at rest; you see the wrinkles when the person is not moving
Early photoaging	Advanced photoaging
Mild pigment changes	Hyperpigmentation
No keratosis	Telangiectasia
Minimal to no wrinkles	Keratosis
Ages 20s–30s or younger	Wrinkles even when not moving
Minimal acne scarring can be seen, if present	Ages 40s–50s
No makeup or minimal makeup necessary	Makeup always worn
	Acne scarring, when present, shows through makeup

Type II	Type IV
Wrinkles only in motion, visible when the person is talking, laughing, frowning, and so on	Wrinkles as predominant characteristic; you see only wrinkles
Early-to-moderate photoaging	Severe photoaging
Lentigines, other pigment	Sallow-ashy skin color
Changes showing	Prior skin cancers
Wrinkles forming	Wrinkles all over
Light keratosis	Makeup not worn, sets in cracks
Nasolabial lines beginning to form	Severe acne scarring
Ages 30s–40s	
Minimal makeup	

rhytids
wrinkles.

elastosis
loss of elasticity; the breakdown of elastin fibers with in the skin.

desquamation
turnover of dead cells. Shedding or peeling of the outermost layer of skin.

Hyperkeratosis
increased build up of dead skin cells.

hyperhydrosis
over hydrated skin.

tactile sensitivity
client feels uncomfortable when certain fabrics or pressures are used on the skin. Even towels can feel uncomfortable.

cosmetic sensitivity
skin that cannot tolerate certain cosmetics, usually fragrances, and preservatives.

environmental sensitivity
irritated easily by sun and wind exposure.

- **Rhytids** (wrinkles)
- **Elastosis** (loss of elasticity)
- Loss of firmness

Keratinization Conditions

This relates to skin that has problems with **desquamation** (dead cell turn over) of the stratum corneum.

- **Hyperkeratosis**—increased roughness in skin, a buildup of dead skin cells

Skin Hydration Conditions

- Dehydration—appears light purple under Woods lamp, parchment paper look
- **Hyperhydrosis**—over-hydrated skin

Skin Sensitivity (Figure 3–3)

- **Tactile sensitivity**—client feels uncomfortable when certain fabrics or pressures are used on the skin. Towels even can feel uncomfortable.
- **Cosmetic sensitivity**—cannot tolerate certain cosmetics, usually fragrances, and preservatives.
- **Environmental sensitivity**—irritated easily by sun and wind exposure.

	Allergies	Irritants
What causes the reaction?	The rejection of a particular substance by the immune system of the body.	A localized irritation caused by a chemical that burns or overexfoliates the skin.
Who has the reaction?	Only people who have a specific allergy to a particular substance.	Any person can have an irritant reaction if enough of the substance comes in contact with the skin.
Can you have the reaction the first time the skin is exposed to a product or chemical?	No.	Yes.
Can the entire body be affected by the reaction?	Yes.	Not usually.
Does the amount of chemical exposure affect the degree of reaction?	Not necessarily. Allergies can occur from a very small amount of exposure.	Yes.
Does the reaction usually occur quickly?	No.	Yes.

Figure 3–3 This chart identifies the cause of a sensitivity to an allergy or irritant.

Step 4: Lifestyle and Health Considerations

It is important for a client intake form to be filled out prior to the skin analysis to determine medications the client takes, illnesses, and lifestyle habits, such as smoking. It is also important to note that although

CONFIDENTIAL SKIN HEALTH SURVEY	
Name: Date:	
Address:	
Phone (H): (C): E-Mail:	
Birthday: ____ / ____ / _____ How did you hear about us?	

Is this your first facial treatment? YES NO	Do you have acne? YES NO
What improvements would you like to see in your skin?	Are you using (or have in the past): Azelex Differin Renova Retin A Tazarac Glycolic or alphahydroxy acids at home? Microdermabrasion? Accutane? If so, when & how long?
Are you currently under a physician's care for a skin condition or other problem? YES NO	Do you experience frequent blemishes? YES NO If so, how frequently?
Are you pregnant? YES NO	Do you have any allergies to food, cosmetics, or drugs? Please list:
Are you taking birth control or hormone replacement therapy? YES NO	Please list current medications:
Do you wear contact lenses? YES NO	What is your current skin care program?
Do you smoke? YES NO	Cleanser:
On a scale of 1 (low) – 10 (high), what is your stress level?	Toner:
Have you had skin cancer? YES NO	Moisturizer:
Please circle if you have the following:	Sunscreen:
	Special treatments:
Asthma Heart problems High/Low Blood Pressure	Have you had any of the following within the last 6 months?
Herpes Sinus Problems	Cosmetic Surgery Laser Resurfacing
Diabetes Epilepsy Frequent Migraines	Chemical Peels Botox
Immune Disorders Metal pins or plates	Restylane or other fillers Microdermabrasion
Thyroid disease Pacemaker Psoriasis	
Have you had permanent cosmetics done? YES NO	Have you had any waxing or electrolysis in the last week? YES NO
I understand that the services offered are not a substitute for medical care, and any information provided will be kept confidential.	
SPA Policies: We require a 24 hour cancellation notice. We do not give cash refunds.	_____ Client Signature

Figure 3–4 A confidential Client Intake Form gives the esthetician the clinical information needed to protect the client while providing services.

Genetic Skin Type				Fitzpatrick Type
Oily	Combination	Normal	Dry	I, II, III, IV, V, VI Circle one

Skin Conditions

Vascular	Lipid System		Pigmentation	Keratin
Telangiectasia	Comedones	Scarred Ostia	Hyperpigmentation	Hyperkeratosis
Diffuse Redness	Seborrhea	Sebaceous Hyperplasia	Hypopigmentation	Skin Hydration
Erythema	Folliculitis		Solar Lentigines	Dehydration
Rosacea	Milia		Melasma	Hyperhydrosis
	Acne I, II, III, IV			

Skin Sensitivity	Aging	Disease or Disorders
Cosmetic Sensitivity	Rubin Type	Rosacea
_____	Glogau Type	Eczema
Tactile Sensitivity	Rhytids	Psoriasis
	Elastosis	Lesions
Environmental Sensitivity		Skin cancer
_____		

Lifestyle
Products used at home   _____

Smokes __yes__no   UV exposure __intermittent __frequently __tanning beds

Recent cosmetic procedures   _____   Medications _____

Treatment Focus	Treatments Given
	Date Type Formula Notes

Figure 3–5 The Client Skin Assessment Form provides a format for recording analysis of the client's skin condition, type, history, and treatment plan.

we are not considered a medical profession, it is wise to comply with HIPAA rules for client confidentiality.

A specific aging treatment consultation could be added to the client consultation to create a comprehensive holistic healthy aging plan. Refer to Figures 3–4 and 3–5 for a client intake form and skin analysis form.

Now, let's put it all together using the skin analysis chart.

Step 1:   Interpret the health questionnaire with your client; focus on the conditions your client feels are most important while noting the inflammatory symptoms that may be present.

Step 2:   Identify the genetic skin type.

Step 3:   Identify the Fitzpatrick skin type or healing response time.

Step 4:   Identify all the conditions within the skin.

Step 5:   Conduct a healthy aging consultation.

Step 6:   Formulate a treatment plan based on the SOAP notes interpretation.

SOAP Notes

SOAP stands for Subjective, Objective, Assessment, and Plan. This system is a medical charting record. For a medical aesthetician this system is required to work with other medical personnel. For an esthetician working in a nonmedical environment this system is not required but is useful for taking all information given by the client and creating an effective treatment program. Let's look at how to modify the SOAP concept to fit esthetic procedures.

Subjective:

Subjective refers to information that your client discloses to you, and is the primary source of lifestyle information. This step requires active listening, which was discussed in Chapter 2. Subjective information is obtained through the intake form as well as verbally. See the client example for subjective information.

> HIPAA stands for the **Health Insurance Portability and Accountability Act**. Title II provides privacy rules which dictate how protected health information (PHI) is used. PHI relates to all aspects of client care, including payment information.

> Health Insurance Portability and Accountability Act (HIPAA)
> legislation that protects the privacy of individually identifiable health information; includes the HIPAA Security Rule, which sets national standards for the security of electronic protected health information; and the confidentiality provisions of the Patient Safety Rule, which protect identifiable information being used to analyze patient safety events and improve patient safety.

Client Example

Let's take the following client example through all steps of the client consult. Here is the pertinent information.

Client: 42-year-old female

Objective of visit: relaxation and wrinkle reduction

Skin care: Concerned with signs of aging: color, texture, wrinkles, and loss of elasticity. The client uses several skin care lines but not consistently and facial treatments several times a year, with Botox® injections twice a year. She thinks her skin is dry and not sensitive and is willing to use multiple products daily.

Lifestyle: Daily fitness routine, takes daily vitamin supplements, moderate drinking, high stress job with frequent travel. Massage as needed.

Health: No major health issues, perimenopausal symptoms, no allergies to products but does have latex sensitivity.

Objective:

This information is based on the estheticians' visual analysis of the skin. Diagnostic tools such as the Woods lamp and magnifying lamp should be used. See steps 1 and 2 for visual signs.

Assessment:

Assessment is based on taking both the subjective and objective information and then correlating it to the tools available to the esthetician. Let's look at our client example, which illustrates both subjective and objective information.

Protocol:

In a normal medical setting this would be Plan, but to modify this system for esthetic practice, protocol is more appropriate. This section of SOAP notes summarizes a comprehensive plan that will be given to the client. This portion of the consultation includes recommendations based on technology and treatments available to the esthetician as well as any professional referrals needed to accomplish

Client Example
Subjective Information:

The following is an example of information disclosed by the client, which would be considered subjective.

Client: 42-year-old female

Objective of visit: relaxation and wrinkle reduction

Skin care: Concerned with signs of aging: color, texture, wrinkles, and loss of elasticity. Uses several skin care lines but not consistently and facial treatments several times a year, with Botox injections twice a year. Thinks her skin is dry and not sensitive and is willing to use multiple products daily.

Lifestyle: Daily fitness routine, supplementation, moderate drinking, high stress job with frequent travel. Massage as needed.

Health: No major health issues, perimenopausal symptoms, no allergies to products but has latex sensitivity.

Objective Information:

The following is considered objective information, which is discovered by the esthetician during an skin assessment.

Skin type: Combination-Fitzpatrick Type 2

Conditions: Photodamage (Rubin type I), dehydration, hyperkeratinization, comedones

Assessment: Client has identified with wrong skin type, thus using the wrong home care products. High stress levels are impacting hydration and texture issues in the skin. Perimenopausal symptoms are adding to the skin condition. Fitzpatrick type is good for most clinical treatments.

the identified goals. If a healthy aging consultation is included in the assessment, this portion would be completed after the client has finished the form. The client example will illustrate how this information is interpreted.

Client Example

Subjective Information:

Client: 42-year-old female

Objective of visit: relaxation and wrinkle reduction

Skin care: Concerned with signs of aging: color, texture, wrinkles, and loss of elasticity. Uses several skin care lines but not consistently and facial treatments several times a year, with Botox injections twice a year. Thinks her skin is dry and not sensitive and is willing to use multiple products daily.

Lifestyle: Daily fitness routine, supplementation, moderate drinking, high stress job with frequent travel. Massage as needed.

Health: No major health issues, perimenopausal symptoms, no allergies to products but has latex sensitivity.

Objective Information:

Skin type: Combination-Fitzpatrick Type 2

Conditions: Photodamage, fine wrinkles (stage 1 aging), dehydration, hyperkeratinization, comedones.

Assessment: Client has identified with wrong skin type thus using the wrong home care products, high stress levels are impacting hydration and texture issues in the skin. Perimenopausal symptoms are adding to skin condition. Fitzpatrick type is good for most clinical treatments.

Lifestyle assessment: Daily fitness is good, diet and water intake may be lacking due to travel and stress. Consistency with self-care and home use of professional products lacking. A program designed around ease of use will be important.

Note: The chapters that follow will continue in detail the options available to treat this client.

The following is an example of the type of interpretation that an esthetician will make after reviewing both subjective and objective information.

Protocols: *Chapter 5 will discuss the next step in our case study.*

Treatments (esthetic and medical): *Outline a plan for at least six months. For example: a series of six glycolic peels and microdermabrasion treatments and three hydrating facials. Be specific for your client and explain the benefits as well as a price. Refer to Chapters 6 and 8 for additional information.*

Home care: *See Chapters 7 for home care guidelines. Always remember to use your manufacturers' guidelines for recommending a home care program.*

Professional service referrals: *List professionals and provide referral information. For example, this client has a high stress level, so recommending a local massage therapist and yoga instructor would be appropriate.*

Lifestyle recommendations: *Professionals can also be used here if the client needs them, for example, a poor diet would benefit from a nutritionist. It is appropriate for an esthetician to recommend lifestyle changes within established guidelines such as fitness, vitamin supplementation, and stress reduction techniques. These are detailed in Chapters 9 to 12.*

The Healthy Aging Consultation

The healthy aging consultation will encompass all aspects of a client's lifestyle as well as attitudes and beliefs about aging. Some manufacturers already have systems in place to support their product line, which can save you time and energy. See Figure 3–6 for an example of a healthy aging consultation form. If you are using a product

AGE POSITIVE CLIENT PROFILE

NAME _____   TODAY'S DATE _____

ADDRESS _____

PHONE _____   ALT. PHONE _____

MY AGE STAGE
☐ Early 20s — 30s
☐ Middle 40s — 50s
☐ Mature 60s and beyond

HOW MY PARENTS AGED

MY MOM   ☐ Great   ☐ Average   ☐ Poorly   MY DAD   ☐ Great   ☐ Average   ☐ Poorly

MY LIFESTYLE

STRESS LEVEL: ☐ high   ☐ medium   ☐ low

EXERCISE: ☐ never   ☐ moderate   ☐ consistent

SMOKER: ☐ yes   ☐ no

DAILY SUN (UV) EXPOSURE _____ (number of hours)

SLEEP: ☐ sufficient   ☐ never enough

DAILY DIET –
  Alcohol: ☐ yes   ☐ no
  Water _____ (glasses per day)
  Coffee _____ (cups per day)

AMOUNT OF TIME I SPEND ON BEAUTY
Skin care _____   makeup _____

I WEAR SUNSCREEN EVERY DAY
☐ yes   ☐ no
If yes, what SPF do you wear _____

THE AGE SIGNS I WOULD LIKE TO ADDRESS

1. DEHYDRATED SKIN
Where do you see this ? _____

2. UNEVEN SKIN TONE
(sun spots, freckles, age spots)
Where do you see this ? _____

3. REDNESS
Where do you see this ? _____

4. DULL, LIFELESS SKIN
Where do you see this ? _____

5. LINES & WRINKLES
Where do you see this ? _____

6. LOSS OF FIRMNESS
Where do you see this ? _____

THE THREE AREAS I WOULD LIKE TO IMPROVE FIRST
1. _____
2. _____
3. _____

MY GOALS FOR LOOKING YOUNGER

☐ I want to look younger now and will do everything I can to make it happen

☐ I want a simple program to improve my appearance, that I can do on a daily basis

☐ I like the way I look now and want to prevent future aging

© BIOELEMENTS®

© 2010 Bioelements/SKU SP720

Figure 3–6 Consultation forms allow you to supply the client with a recommended regimen to help achieve their anti-aging goals.

manufacturer who does not utilize a consultation such as this, here are questions to address:

- What signs of aging are you concerned about? Loss of firmness, wrinkles, discolorations, etc.
- What is your current skin care routine?
- How much time do you spend on skin care and makeup daily?
- Do you get regular esthetic treatments or massage?
- Do you get regular medical esthetic treatments or injections?
- Are you using any topical pharmaceutical products, such as Retin-A®, Latisse®, Refirme™, Metrogel®?
- What is your daily fitness routine?
- What are your daily activities—office work, housework, outside work environment?
- Do you smoke?

    - How much per day?

- How much alcohol do you drink?
- Have you experienced menopause (surgical or natural)?
- Do you take hormone replacement therapy?
- Do you use daily UV protection?
- Do you use tanning beds?
- Do you experience chronic pain?
- Do you have any medical disorders?
- Does your weekly diet consist of the following:

    - Processed food
    - Soda and caffeine
    - High protein
    - High fat
    - Vegetables
    - Fish
    - Nuts
    - Supplements such as multivitamins, vitamin D3, and essential fatty acids

- What is your stress level?

    - High
    - Moderate
    - Low

- Have you experienced any major life changes within the last two years?

All of these questions are important to creating an effective program. The consultation may seem in-depth, but each question has a direct correlation to how you treat a client's skin (Figure 3–7).

Question	Interpretation
• What signs of aging are you concerned about? I.e., loss of firmness, wrinkles, discolorations, etc.	Focus on the initial signs of aging that the client is concern with, and then build a program around all other conditions found.
• What is your current skin care routine?	If the client is only using two products twice a day, the at-home program must be simple. Explain the fact that a limited result will be found if the client cannot comply with at-home and professional treatments.
• How much time do you spend on skin care and makeup daily?	Test the pH of cleansers and treatment products; a prolonged alkaline pH of the skin will lead to TEWL, which affects all enzyme processes within the skin.
• Do you get regular esthetic treatments or massage?	Knowing a client's level of professional care will help determine how quickly improvements can be seen.
• Do you get regular medical esthetic treatments or injections?	An esthetician must know about all injectable fillers and other noninvasive treatment in order to design a safe program. No facial treatments 72 hours after Botox® or fillers. Microcurrent will not work over areas that have Botox®.
• Are you using any topical pharmaceutical products? I.e., Retin-A, Latisse, ReFirme, Metrogel, etc.	Many professional products cannot be combined with pharmaceutical products. Best to focus on barrier repair to reduce side effects of many prescription treatments.
• What is your daily fitness routine?	One of the quickest areas to improve the skin. Should be emphasized with every client.
• What are your daily activities? I.e., office work, housework, outside work environment, etc.	This will determine the level of UVR protection needed daily.
• Do you smoke? • How much per day?	Very hard to improve the skin with a smoker. Amount per day will help determine the type of professional treatments to use. For example, a light smoker may handle a light AHA peel better than a heavy smoker.
• How much alcohol do you drink?	This relates to level of chronic inflammation that may be present as well as increased dehydration in skin.
• Have you experienced menopause (surgical or natural)?	Menopause has a direct effect on the skin regardless of the type, surgical or natural. This also gives the client a chance to talk about hormone replacement therapy, which is important to address.
• Do you take hormone replacement therapy?	HRT does improve the signs of aging. Natural therapies are available as well.
• Do you use daily UV protection?	#1 aging preventer. Opening the dialog for appropriate daily protection application, etc.

Figure 3–7 A healthy aging consult chart helps interpret answers clients provide.

Question	Interpretation
• Do you use tanning beds?	Same side effects as smoking, unable to improve skin while client is doing this. Can help protect the skin and the client, though.
• Do you experience chronic pain?	Chronic pain can indicate chronic subclinical inflammation. Important that the source is addressed.
• Do you have any medical disorders?	This is a sensitive subject for clients; estheticians need to know about diabetes (slow healing), heart disease (chronic inflammation), blood disorders (possible Coumadin use), asthma (careful with steam), fibromyalgia (discomfort on table), cancer (skin can be over sensitive from treatment), as well as other conditions
• Does your weekly diet consist of the following: • Processed food • Soda / caffeine • High protein • High fat • Vegetables • Fish • Nuts • Supplements such as multivitamin, vitamin D3, essential fatty acids	Diet directly relates to the condition of the skin. Processed food leads to increased glycation and inflammation within the body. Loss of elasticity may be apparent with a high fatty, sugar diet. Acne is aggravated by iodine. Lack of vitamin D is known to impact the immune system. Increasing a clients' vitamin D3 intake can help improve rosacea and other disorders.
• What is your stress level? • High • Moderate • Low	High stress levels increase amount of cortisol within the body, which leads to weight gain and increased inflammation and glycation. The body's ability to withstand free radicals is also decreased, leading to cellular damage.
• Have you experienced major life changes within the last two years?	This indicates a client's chronic stress level. Death, moving, and financial troubles can cause long-term chronic stress. This client needs a safe quiet place to be, with a focus on stress reduction through touch.

Figure 3–7 Continued.

■ CREATING A TEAM OF PROFESSIONALS

A team of professionals is important for designing an effective healthy aging treatment program. A team of professionals will also help you market your services by creating a referral network, and offer effective treatment options for the client. Estheticians have a specific scope of practice and unless they are trained in other fields, they will need an educated expert to help support the client.

Board certifications are confusing. The bottom line is that the American Board of Medical Specialties (ABMS) oversees 24 subspecialties in medicine, which include dermatology and plastic surgery. The only plastic surgery board accepted by ABMS is the American Board of Plastic Surgery. In order to become certified by the American Board of Plastic Surgery, a surgeon must first complete an approved residency in plastic surgery, pass a written qualifying examination, and then an oral certifying examination.

There are other boards that certify as well, but they are not accepted by the American Board of Medical Specialties. One of these other boards is the American Society of Plastic Surgeons, which requires six years of experience with three in plastic surgery. The bottom line is finding out where the doctor is certified and what the requirements are before recommending their services.

Here are some of the experts who can help:

- *Nutritionist*: basic nutrition information can be passed on by the esthetician to the client, but an in-depth nutritional plan is valuable for improving general health and preventing many different problems with the skin. Many physical problems can be corrected with improvement in dietary habits.
- *Therapist*: mental stress causes direct physical symptoms. Many issues arise when dealing with aging issues, such as grief, loss of self-esteem, chronic pain, and feelings of isolation. A therapist can help give a client an outlet with professional guidance to correct the issues that cannot be addressed in the treatment room.
- *Fitness expert*: fitness is one of the most effective ways to improve the skin. It has a direct impact on the skin and general well-being. Being physically fit slows the aging process and has many benefits. Having an expert for your client to see can increase motivation and provide results that a self-directed program may miss.
- *Massage therapist*: chronic pain causes chronic inflammation which directly affects the aging process, and massage can make a difference in how a client feels. Many estheticians are also licensed massage therapists, which is a perfect complement.
- *Dermatologist and plastic surgeon*: abnormalities in the skin appear with aging clientele, and a dermatological referral can be invaluable. Plastic surgeons are valuable for clients who have advanced dermal aging issues that an esthetician may not treat. Many have estheticians on staff, which could cause a conflict, so check your referrals out closely. Asking colleagues and clients who have had good experiences is a great resource. Make sure they are board certified.
- *Naturopathic physician*: many clients prefer a natural approach to healthcare and many estheticians have had personal experience with this healthcare approach and have seen results with stubborn skin conditions that do not respond to an allopathic medical approach. These physicians are licensed by the state they work in, and education requirements are stringent.
- *Hairstylist*: a good hair color treatment and haircut can take years off. This is an excellent complement to an esthetic practice.
- *Makeup artist* (estheticians are also trained in makeup): an outdated application of makeup can add the appearance of years. Just changing the color of a makeup base and teaching a client to contour the face can take years off.

The way to reach these experts depends on the area that the esthetician is living in. Professionals can be people that the esthetician has personally used or clients have recommended.

How to Set up the Network of Professionals

1. Create an initial meeting with your potential professional; note how the expert runs his or her business. Explain clearly why you are calling and what you would like from them. Be prepared that a dermatologist or plastic surgeon may not offer to meet with you.
2. Bring all printed material to the meeting and offer the expert a free treatment and samples of products to get them comfortable with the services offered.
3. Ask for printed material from the expert to distribute to clients.
4. Talk to your professional about any special offers that they may have to extend to your clients and what you would be willing to offer their clients.
5. Check in monthly to follow up on any referrals given or give feedback from clients.

◉ ▪ HANDLING LIABILITY ISSUES

Occasionally there is a break down in communication, mistaken skin assessment occurs, or the unfortunate incidence of a client looking for compensation can come up. As more and more of the medical community becomes involved in esthetics and the technology becomes more invasive, the risk of liability issues increases. The importance of professional liability insurance cannot be overemphasized.

A liability issue can be something as simple as clients unhappy with their results and wanting a refund, or as complicated as a client who wants to sue the esthetician because of damage to the skin.

Causes for Estheticians Being Faced with Liability Issues

- Unrealistic expectations
- Undisclosed health issues
- Nondisclosure of lifestyle choices such as smoking, tanning, and drug use
- Noncompliance with home care recommendations and treatment schedules
- Incorrect skin assessment
- Poor training on manufacturer protocols and ingredients

Avoiding Liability

The following are guidelines for avoiding liability issues:

- General consent forms with health history
- Chemical and advanced procedure informed consent forms as well as liability waivers
- Clearly written post-care instructions
- In-depth manufacturer training as well as manuals with clear written directions
- Consistent advanced education in the science of the skin, cosmetic chemistry, and advanced procedures
- Clear client documentation, such as photos and SOAP notes

What to Do When a Situation Occurs

In the treatment room, clients could encounter a reaction to products. In this situation, you should:

- Have products available specifically for soothing the skin such as colloidal oatmeal, aloe vera, hydrocortisone, gel masks, or what your manufacturer recommends.
- Contact the manufacturer immediately via phone.
- Document the phone call and instructions given.

Symptoms resulting from treatment most commonly occur after the client goes home. Here are some steps to follow:

Your liability insurance provider should give you guidelines for dealing with different situations. Always follow their directions.

When to recommend a visit to a physician?

- Abnormal swelling
- Blisters
- Severe client discomfort
- Bleeding
- Trouble breathing

- Document the conversation. This can be done while on the phone or immediately after.
- Document the description of the problem, symptoms experienced, and advice given.
- Schedule a follow-up appointment as soon as possible. If the client declines, recommend that they see a physician if symptoms do not improve. Take photos if client does come in, and document objective observations. Offering a refund should be based on company policy and how treatment procedures were followed. It is generally a good idea to provide a refund in order to avoid a negative reputation if miscommunication by the esthetician was at the heart of the problem.
- Contact your liability insurance company if the client requests payment for damage to the skin, or threatens to sue.
- Contact the manufacturer of the products or technology used during treatment. Inform them of the situation and ask for advice.

How to Deal with It

When a situation leaves a client upset or with damage to the skin, the esthetician is also impacted. The stress can be detrimental and if it is traumatic enough, motivation to stay within the esthetic profession can be diminished. Here are some guidelines that may help the esthetician through a difficult time.

- Do not take it personally; often the client's attack is not on the esthetician. A client's motivation rarely takes into account anyone else around them. Try to be as objective as possible.
- Talk to someone. Having a support system is important when dealing with a stressful situation. This is not gossip; find someone who is objective and not involved in the situation.
- Contact your insurance adjuster. Speaking to someone who has the facts of the situation can alleviate speculation and fear. Get the facts.
- Limit verbal and written communication with the client.
- Analyze what happened. Every situation is a learning experience, even one that may not be the esthetician's fault.

> > > **Top Ten Tips to Take to the Clinic**

1. Always start a healthy aging consult with correct skin assessment.
2. Remember that the color of the skin is not always an indicator of how the skin will respond to treatment.
3. Always ask about healing response time.
4. Lifestyle questions are important to the outcome of the plan.
5. Be knowledgeable about the medical procedures available for the client even if they are out of your scope of practice.
6. Understand the basic skin types and visual clues.
7. Always take SOAP notes, as this will improve the treatment outcome.
8. Prevent liability situations by always doing a health intake form.
9. Set up a network of professionals to help you grow.
10. Have a plan to deal with a liability issue if it happens.

Chapter Review Questions

1. What should you do if a liability situation occurs during a treatment?

2. What are the characteristics of dry skin?

3. What are the characteristics of oily skin?

4. What are the characteristics of combination skin?

5. What questions should you ask your client to determine a client's healing response time?

Bibliography

Baumann, L. MD., Saghari, S. MD., Weisburg, E. MS., (2009). *Cosmetic Dermatology: Principles and Practice*, 2nd Edition. New York: McGraw-Hill Medical.

Culp, J., et al. (2010). *Milady's Standard Esthetics: Advanced*, 1st Edition. Clifton Park, NY: Cengage Learning.

Lees, Mark P.H.D. (2001). *Skin Care: Beyond the Basics*. New York: Thomson Delmar Learning.

Michalun, N., Michalun, M. V. (2010). *Milady's Skin Care and Cosmetic Ingredients Dictionary*, 3rd Edition. Clifton Park, NY: Cengage Learning.

Nordman, L. (2005). *Professional Beauty Therapy: The Official Guide to Level 3*, 2nd ed. London: Thomson Learning.

Schmaling, S. (2008). *Milady's Aesthetician Series: A Comprehensive Guide to Equipment*. Clifton Park, NY: Cengage Learning.

Websites

http://www.ascpskincare.com
http://www.bioelements.com

What Happens When We Age?

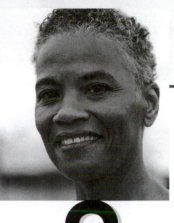

Section **2**

Basics of Aging

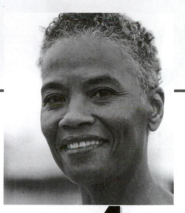

Chapter 4

Key Terms

adenosine triphosphate (ATP)

alveoli

calcium pump protein

chromosomes

CRP (C-reactive protein)

extrinsic aging

free radicals

gerontology

IL-6

intrinsic aging

macro aging

micro aging

mitral valve

nucleic acids

phagocytes

reactive oxygen species (ROS)

SA node

senescence

somatic cells

telomerase

telomeres

tumor necrosis factor-alpha

ventricular walls

Learning Objectives

After completing this chapter, you will be able to:

1. Describe the currently accepted theories on aging.
2. Recognize the signs of aging in cells, organs, and body systems.

▪ INTRODUCTION: THEORIES OF AGING

It seems that clients are always trying to find the next anti-aging miracle treatment, whereas estheticians are trying to meet their needs by attempting anything that sounds plausible. This usually brings up more questions than answers. To be successful in esthetics, a basic knowledge of why we age and the hypothesis behind the science is helpful. One of the many questions asked is whether aging is a disease or an inevitable process that all biological creatures must experience, or can it be prevented?

This is the central question that is the focus in the science of **senescence**. Senescence is the term used to refer to the biological process of aging and is used to define an entire body of scientific study. **Gerontology** is another subspecialty of medicine that focuses on the study, treatment, and management of aging. Senescence or aging manifests in many ways within the human body. In general, the process of aging creates increased intolerance to stress, increased imbalance in body systems, and increased risk to age-related diseases.

Estheticians often refer to the intrinsic and extrinsic types of aging. This is a simplified description and requires more in-depth explanation. **Intrinsic aging** defines the internal signs of aging as a genetic process, and **extrinsic aging** refers to the visible signs of aging caused by external lifestyle factors. These internal and external factors directly relate to two separate groups of aging theories, preprogrammed and damage-based theories. Different ways to describe aging signs are macro and micro aging. **Macro aging** refers to the signs of aging that are visible. **Micro aging** refers to the aging that is happening at the cellular level. When micro aging accumulates over time it then becomes macro, or visible signs of damage.

It is important to note that preprogrammed and damage-based theories influence each other. In esthetics we focus mainly on the damage-based theories due to the fact that we can control some of the damage that can happen, but technology is rapidly advancing to influence how we can also influence genetic cellular aging. In this chapter we will explore both programmed and damaged-based theories of aging.

It is also important to note that these theories are all hypotheses. These hypotheses are a small representation of the scientific work happening in the study of aging. At this time scientists cannot agree on the causes of aging or if it is an inevitable process we all must go through.

Programmed Theories

Programmed theories of aging refer to aging that is due to genetic factors. This category of theory suggests that aging is determined by a

senescence
process of cell aging.

gerontology
the scientific study of the biological, psychological, and sociological phenomena associated with old age and aging.

intrinsic aging
aging that is influenced by genetics.

extrinsic aging
visible signs of aging caused by external lifestyle factors.

macro aging
refers to the signs of aging that are visible.

micro aging
refers to the aging that is happening at the cellular level.

predetermined biological clock started at conception, that genes play a strong role in the aging process, and certain genetic factors such as defensive or protective genes impact how the individual ages. There are several accepted theories that focus on the genetic causes of aging, including those outlined in the sections that follow.

Programmed Longevity Theory

The programmed longevity theory is also known as the Hayflick theory, named for the scientist Leonard Hayflick. The focus of the theory is that cells divide a set number of times before they die. Hayflick was able to prove that a cell can divide only 50 times before death and that nutrition will have a direct effect on cell division, with underfed cells dividing more slowly than overfed cells. This theory has led directly to the calorie restriction lifestyle to slow cell death.

Telomerase Theory

Recently a new theory has been posed regarding DNA damage called the telomerase theory of aging. **Telomerase** is an enzyme involved in the repair and replacement of shortened telomeres. **Telomeres** are sequences of **nucleic acids** that extend to form the ends of **chromosomes**. They have no genetic function but act as protection for the chromosome. Telomeres are critical for healthy cellular function. See Figure 4–1 for an example of a telomere.

The telomeres shorten each time a cell divides, which leads to cellular damage due to the cell not being able to duplicate itself correctly. Each time this damaged cell duplicates itself it becomes worse, and eventually dies. This leads to cellular dysfunction, aging, and death.

telomerase
an enzyme that adds DNA sequence.

telomeres
region of repetitive DNA at the end of a chromosome, which protects the end of the chromosome from deterioration.

nucleic acids
any of a group of complex compounds found in all living cells and viruses, composed of purines, pyrimidines, carbohydrates, and phosphoric acid. Nucleic acids in the form of DNA and RNA control cellular function and heredity.

chromosomes
organized structure of DNA and protein found within cells.

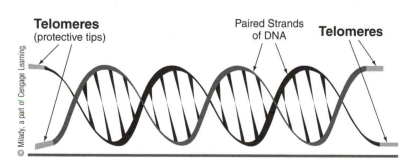

CHROMOSOMES ARE PAIRED STRANDS OF DNA FORMED AS THE DOUBLE HELIX

Telomeres (protective tips)

Paired Strands of DNA

Telomeres

© Milady, a part of Cengage Learning.

Figure 4–1 An example of a telomere, described in the telomerase theory.

In August 2000, *Experimental Cell Research* published a study by W. Funk et al.[1] that has shown that by inducing the human telomere gene (hTERT) into in vitro aging skin, damage associated with aging skin is reversed. This includes increased fibroblasts and overall improved skin function. This research has opened the door for the possibility of topical treatments that would insert the human telomere gene into the epidermis to reset gene expression. Currently this type of work is being conducted on several groups of people. One of those groups is children with progeria, a disease that causes substantial premature aging and death.

It is important to note that there is some discussion about the effectiveness of telomerase gene therapy and if it may induce tumor growth. Telomerase is found in cancer cells and is dormant in normal adult cells. Telomerase is the number one target for chemotherapy due to the cells, ability to reactivate telomerase expression.

Pacemaker Theory

The pacemaker theory is also referred to as the rate of living theory. This theory suggests that we have a finite number of breaths or that our hearts beat a predetermined number of times. Modern scientists have found that a more plausible model for this theory is the rate that oxygen is metabolized by the body. This is based on the observation that animals with rapid metabolisms tend to have the shortest life spans. This hypothesis was created by Raymond Pearl in 1928 and is considered a flawed theory.

Genetic Theory

The genetic theory is also recognized as a planned obsolescence theory. This theory focuses on programming encoded within our DNA. DNA (Figure 4–2) is considered the blueprint of life that we inherit from our parents. Each person is born with a unique code; this indicates a predetermined tendency for certain types of diseases, physical and mental functioning, appearance, and regulating the rate at which we age.

Even though this theory is thought of as a preprogrammed theory, it has been proven that environmental damage can influence how a person ages due to the damage that DNA can suffer. We have the ability to impact the amount of DNA damage by our lifestyle choices.

Immunological Theory

Included in this category is the immunological theory. This theory states that the immune system is designed to decline over time. Starting before age 20 the thymus begins to shrink, which leads to a reduction in T cells. When T cells diminish, protection and tissue repair also decrease. Over time the immune system cannot protect the body from

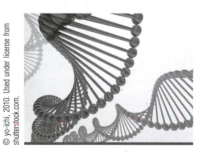

Figure 4–2 An example of DNA, described in the genetic theory.

bacteria, viruses, or toxins, or identify and remove cancer cells. Although the reduction in immune response occurs over time, it is unlikely to be the primary cause of aging.

Somatic Mutation Theory

Somatic mutation theory, suggested by Leo Szilard in 1958, states that the chromosomes inherited from our parents can affect our life span, primarily based on mutations that the parent has acquired through exposure to ionizing radiation. This theory further states that **somatic cells** can be damaged by UV radiation and environmental toxins and create genetic mutations over time which would lead to an accelerated rate of aging. An analogy often used is that each time a cell divides a copy of DNA is made, and over time you get errors, just like using a photocopier to duplicate an original document and then copying the copy.

Damaged-based Theories

Damage-based theories refer to aging that is influenced by environmental or lifestyle factors that cause damage to cells and body systems. These theories focus on the damage that happens at the molecular level and then move outward. To understand the concept of damage-based theories it is important to understand what a free radical is and how it can affect the life of a cell.

The basic building block of the cell is the atom. An atom consists of the nucleus, protons, electrons, and neutrons (Figure 4–3). The number of protons determines the number of electrons orbiting the nucleus. Electrons hold atoms together to make a molecule and orbit the atom in one or more shells. The inner shell is full when it has two paired electrons. When the first shell is full then electrons move to the second shell, always balancing their numbers. The number of electrons in its outer shell determines the chemical behavior of an atom. An atom will always try to sustain maximum stability and will do this by gaining or losing electrons and/or bonding with other atoms. See Figure 4–4 for diagram of molecule.

Molecules in turn create cells. **Free radicals** are created at the molecular level and then when the damage is not repaired it affects a living cell. The term *free radical* describes any molecule that has one or more unpaired electrons that can exist independently and react with a healthy molecule in a destructive way.[2] The goal of an atom is to always be balanced and a free radical molecule has an extra electron that creates an extra negative charge. This causes it to bind itself to another balanced molecule as it tries to steal electrons. The balanced molecule then becomes a free radical itself (Figure 4–5 A and B).

somatic cells
one of the cells that take part in the formation of the body.

free radicals
an atom or group of atoms that has at least one unpaired electron and is therefore unstable and highly reactive. Free radicals can damage cells and are believed to accelerate the progression of cancer, cardiovascular disease, and age-related diseases.

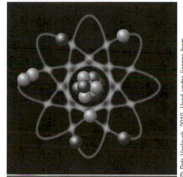

Figure 4–3 An atom is the basic building block of cells.

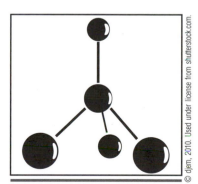

Figure 4–4 A molecule is part of the cellular makeup.

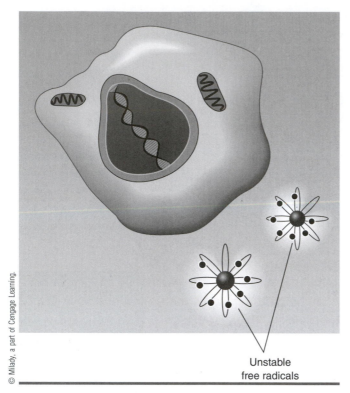

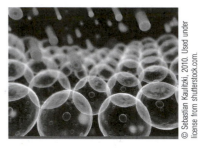

Figure 4–5 Examples of a free radical, which creates damage to cells.

reactive oxygen species (ROS)

term used to describe free radicals due to the fact that most significant free radicals are oxygen centered

Free radical damage is also known as oxidative damage. **Reactive oxygen species (ROS)** is another term used to describe free radicals due to the fact that most significant free radicals are oxygen centered, but not all ROS can be considered free radicals. Hydrogen peroxide is an example of an ROS that is not considered a free radical, but it can be dangerous to a cell. An ROS is a small molecule that includes oxygen ions, is very reactive, and is formed as a natural by-product of oxygen. One electron reduction of oxygen results in forming reactive oxygen species. This means that when a molecule accepts an oxygen atom, it becomes unstable.

The body also produces free radicals naturally. This is the result of natural body processes such as:

- Breathing. Oxygen is a potent free radical accelerator.
- Inflammatory immune response. Phagocytosis, inflammation, and apoptosis are all important in this chemistry. Phagocytosis is the cellular process of engulfing solid particles for ingestion. From this process inflammation is created and then apoptosis or cell death occurs.

- Production of energy within the mitochondria. When **ATP (adenosine triphosphate)**, the universal energy molecule used by the body, is produced, free radicals are released.

When ROS are created they can attack the structure of cell membranes. This process creates metabolic waste. A toxic accumulation of this waste interferes with cellular communication, alters DNA and RNA, and disrupts protein synthesis. This leads to lower energy levels, which impedes vital chemical cellular processes. The membrane theory of aging explores this phenomenon.

Multiple types of free radicals are generated within the body. They are singlet oxygen, superoxide radical, lipid peroxide, hydrogen peroxide, and hydroxyl radical. Each one damages the cell in different ways. See Table 4–1 chart of free radical damage.

The most damaging free radicals are the hydroxyl radical and the superoxide radical. Not all antioxidants will neutralize these free radicals. If an ineffective antioxidant is used, higher damage producing free radicals will be converted into a greater number of lower damage producing free radicals. This leads to increased damage.

A healthy body can naturally neutralize the free radicals, but a body under stress must have help to neutralize them. The damage that free radicals cause can be minimized by antioxidants known as

ATP (adenosine triphosphate)
this molecule provides cellular energy transport and enzyme regulation.

Types of free radicals:
Singlet oxygen–created by UV radiation; indoor fluorescent lighting is strong enough to induce in skin.[2]
Superoxide radial–attacks enzymes and cell membrane, promotes the creation of lipofuscin.
Lipid peroxide–oxidizes cell membrane and barrier lipids; inflammation.
Hydrogen peroxide–present when inflammation occurs; can be converted to hydroxyl radical when exposed to iron; diffuses across cell membranes.
Hydroxyl radical–most damaging radical; attacks and kills or mutates all DNA; attacks all parts of cell; causes cross linking.

Table 4–1 A chart describing damage caused by different types of free radicals.

Free Radical Type	Damage Created
Superoxide Radical	• Attacks enzymes and cell membrane • Promotes creation of lipofuscin • Activates enzymes that break down cell lipids/arachidonic acid
Hydrogen Peroxide	• Can be converted to hydroxyl radical when exposed to iron, diffuses across cell membranes
Hydroxyl Radical	• Most dangerous, attacks all parts of cell • Causes cross linking • Activate transcription factors NF-kB (proinflammatory), AP-1 (microscarring) • Cell death and injury • DNA destruction
Singlet Oxygen	• Created by UV radiation • Cell death and injury

free radical scavengers. Antioxidants will bind to free radicals and help stabilize them.

The first line of defense against ROS within the body is three antioxidant enzymes:

- Superoxide dismutase—first to respond; converts ROS to hydrogen peroxide.
- Catalase—converts hydrogen peroxide to water and oxygen.
- Glutathione peroxidase—works with catalase to convert hydrogen peroxide to water and oxygen.

These enzymes are naturally produced within the body, stop ROS, and then convert them to harmless substances such as water.

The second line of defense is the lipid and water soluble antioxidants. Some of these can be taken internally via food or supplementation.

Lipid Soluble Antioxidants

- Vitamin E (tocopherol)
- Beta carotene (provitamin A)
- CoQ10 (Ubiquinol, ubiquinone)

Water Soluble Antioxidants

- Vitamin C (ascorbic acid)
- Glutathione
- Uric acid

It is recommended that a blend of multiple antioxidants be taken internally to minimize free radical damage. The blend can include beta carotene, vitamin C, grape seed extract, and vitamin E. This can be taken via supplementation or more effectively in a balanced diet.

Free radical damage is considered a factor in many diseases, such as cancer, arthritis, atherosclerosis, Alzheimer's disease, and diabetes. This link has been made due to the chemical processes that happen within the cell due to free radicals.

> You should note that it is dangerous to use lipid soluble vitamin supplementation, especially vitamin E, in excess. It is recommended not to exceed the 400 IU a day for vitamin E and 10,000 IU a day for vitamin A. Lipid soluble vitamins are not easily eliminated by the body as they are stored in fat cells.

Free Radical Theory

This is the most widely accepted theory of aging and was developed by Denham Harman, MD, in 1956 at the University of Nebraska. Dr. Harman's theory states that aging is caused by accumulated free radicals attacking the DNA, proteins, and fats of a living cell, causing cell death. Dr. Harman further expanded his theory in 1972 to state that the part of the cell most sensitive to damage was the mitochondria. He also theorized that a nontoxic dose of antioxidants and other nutrients could slow the aging process within the mitochondria.

It has been proven that lifestyle and environment can accelerate free radical production in the body. The factors that accelerate the creation of free radicals within the environment and lifestyle of an individual are:

- Smoking
- Exposure to radiation (UVA and UVB)
- Chronic stress
- Excessive alcohol consumption
- Drugs
- Lack of sleep

The Membrane Theory of Aging

The membrane theory was created by Imre Zs-Nagy, professor of Debrecen University in Hungary. This theory states that it is the damage done by free radicals in the cells' membrane that causes changes in the cells' ability to transfer chemicals, heat, and electricity, which leads to cellular damage and thus aging. With aging, the cell membrane becomes less permeable and more solid. This causes the cell to lose its efficiency to conduct normal functions. This includes a reduction in the transfer of sodium and potassium, which impairs cellular communication. This will lead to toxic accumulation and cell death.

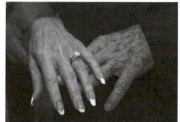

Figure 4–6 Lipofuscin is responsible for age-related pigmentation problems.

The toxin that is accumulated is called lipofuscin and is responsible for age-related pigmentation problems such as liver spots (Figure 4–6). Lipofuscin deposits are also found in the brain, lungs, and heart as a person ages. It has been theorized that this can contribute to Alzheimer's disease, and indeed Alzheimer's patients have been tested to show that they have a much higher rate of lipofuscin deposits than a healthy person.

The Cross Linking Theory

The cross linking theory of aging is also referred to as the glycation theory. This theory relates to the binding of protein and simple sugars (glucose) to protein. This happens when oxygen is present. When cross linking occurs, protein is damaged and unable to perform as intended. We see this as thick, dry, sagging, and yellow skin. It is also known that free radicals can lead to cross linking.

Cross linking is responsible for many age-related disorders:

- **Diabetes**. Often viewed as a form of accelerated aging, diabetes is the imbalance of insulin and glucose tolerance. It has been found that diabetics have two to three times the number of cross linked proteins as a nondiabetic.

- **Cardiac enlargement**. Cross linked proteins harden collagen, which makes the heart more susceptible to cardiac arrest.
- **Renal disorders**. Kidneys have inside them tiny structures called nephrons that filter blood. They remove waste products and water. Cross linking can damage the nephrons, resulting in kidney disease.
- **Cancer**. It is theorized that sugars binding to DNA may cause malformed cells that can lead to cancer.
- **Senile cataracts**. This is a vision-impairing disease that is caused by the thickening of the lens in the eye. Cross linked proteins can lead to this thickening.

The Mitochondrial Theory

Mitochondria are organelles found in every cell. They are responsible for producing energy. The goal of the mitochondria is to produce ATP (adenosine triphosphate), the fuel that every cell in our body uses. Every thought, action, and movement we make is the result of ATP within the cell. Little ATP can be stored within the body, and reserves of ATP are no more than 5 ounces. The mitochondria must be healthy to supply the body with the continuous supply of ATP needed for the repair and regenerative processes to occur. Mitochondria are exposed to a large amount of free radical damage and do not have the same defenses found throughout the body.

This leads to a reduction in ATP production that affects how the organs function. When an organ's mitochondria fail, that particular organ's function and repair processes are impacted, which could lead to disease and death.

Neuroendocrine Theory

The neuroendocrine theory, which was proposed by Vladimir Dilman and Ward Dean MD, indicates that wear and tear on this system accelerates the aging process. The neuroendocrine system is governed by the hypothalamus, a walnut-sized gland located in the brain. The hypothalamus regulates a network of biochemicals that trigger the release of hormones. This leads to various reactions that instruct the organs and glands to release hormones that control the function of the body. The hypothalamus also monitors and responds to the levels of hormones within each organ and gland.

With age, the hypothalamus loses its ability to regulate hormones with precision. The uptake receptors also become less sensitive to hormones. This results in a decline in the production and effectiveness of certain hormones as we age.

The loss of regulation may be attributed to damage caused to the hypothalamus by the hormone cortisol. Cortisol is considered the stress hormone; it is produced by the adrenal glands located above the kidneys. This is the one hormone that increases with age. Chronic unresolved stress both physical and mental can cause an abundance of cortisol within the body, which can lead to increased damage to the hypothalamus as well as other organs. When cortisol damages the hypothalamus, cortisol production is increased, which leads to more damage again. It can be a never-ending cycle.

Wear and Tear Theory

The wear and tear theory was suggested in 1882 by August Weismann. This theory states that somatic cells cannot repair themselves, so over time wear and tear creates damage that causes aging and death. This is the beginning of aging theory that led to the free radical and cross linking theories.

New Hypotheses

New hypotheses of aging are being introduced all the time. The current newly released theories are:

Inflammation Theory

The inflammation theory of aging states that the long-term effects of chronic inflammation result in accumulated damage to the body. This theory may explain the cause of many diseases and disorders such as:

- Alzheimer's
- Atherosclerosis
- Osteoporosis
- Depression
- Diabetes

Inflammation is one of the immune responses that can help protect us from invaders and traumatic events. Take for example the instance of a cut. First, coagulation begins to slow down the bleeding and prevent germs from spreading. Then **phagocytes**, cells that swallow and destroy pathogens, merge upon the damage. These phagocytes secrete cytokines, messenger proteins, which call for more responders. Phagocytes also create ROS, which will also destroy bacteria. Throughout the body other chemical reactions are taking place at the same time via other cytokines such as **IL-6, tumor necrosis factor-alpha**, and **CRP (C-reactive protein)**, which will eliminate remaining bacteria. This is a specialized adaptive immune response called the immune cascade. See Table 4–2 for a chart of the immune cascade.

phagocytes
white blood cells that protect the body by ingesting (phagocytosing) harmful foreign particles, bacteria, and dead or dying cells.

Table 4–2 A chart detailing the immune cascade, the body's response to bacteria.

Step 1 Invasion of Foreign Antibodies	Invaders are recognized by area infiltrated and type of invader determines response.	
1a. Macrophages will respond first if area invaded is primarily defended by them. Example: lungs and intestine	1b. Bacteria such as staph invade and produce chemotaxins, which immediately activate phagocytes.	1c. Other bacteria invade and are recognized by the complement system, which in turn produces cytokines that start the immune response.
	1d. Lymphocytes directly fight invader or control other cells when recognized by acquired immune system (humeral immune system).	
Step 2 Immune Cascade	Phagocytes move to site of invasion and activate, which produces cytokines.	
Step 3 Cytokines Activate	Cytokines (chemical messengers) cause cells to perform certain immune functions.	

Cytokine	Cell	Actions
Interleukin-1	Macrophages	Acts to initiate inflammation, increases body temperature via the hypothalamus
Interleukin-2, 3, 4, 5, 6, 10,12,13	T Cells & some Macrophages	Increases immune cells and induces antibody destruction, creates growth of immune cells in bone marrow, promotes B cell growth, some activation of macrophages, ILK10 inhibits macrophages
Gamma-Interferon	T Cells, NK Cells	Activates macrophages
Tumor Necrosis Factor (TNF)	Macrophages	Induces inflammation, fever, catabolism of muscle and fat
Transforming Growth Factor (TGF)	T Cells, Macrophages	Inhibits T cell growth and macrophage activation
Lymphotoxin	T Cells	Activates macrophages

Step 4 Blood Circulation Increases	Blood vessels dilate, gaps appear within cell walls surrounding invasion, which allows larger immune cells to pass through. Histamine is released, which induces blood vessel dilation and permeability. Increased body heat and proteins. Phagocytes continue to destroy and digest invaders.	
Step 5 Inflammation Ends	Apoptosis signal is received from Helper T cells. If T cells do not recognize antigen destruction, chronic inflammation can develop.	

The effects of the inflammatory response are varied but all important when activated for a short term. They are as follows:

- Blood circulation increases around the affected area.
- Channels appear in the cell walls, allowing larger immune cells to pass through.
- Immune cells and proteins surround the site and strengthen the immune response. This leads to swelling within the tissue.
- An increase in body heat has an antibiotic effect. The tissue in the area of damage will become red and warm.
- The area of damage can become painful from expansion of tissues as well as pain mediators.

Once this inflammation cascade is started it should end when the infection is gone. The problem comes when the immune response is activated without an invader or does not receive the signal from helper T cells that tells the immune cells to stop.

The method that the body uses to stop the inflammation cascade is not clearly known. What is known is that one of the mechanisms used is apoptosis. Apoptosis is a chemical signal that tells the cell to kill itself. Some cells, such as immune cells, are designed to use apoptosis within a certain amount of time, but when they are given a message to *stay alive* they do not commit apoptosis until the message is no longer received. The T cells from the immune system emit the *stay alive* message as long as a foreign antibody is recognized by the immune system. When the T cells do not recognize that the antibody has been removed, then chronic inflammation begins.

Atherosclerosis is an example of the chronic inflammation process. When fatty deposits build up in the arteries, macrophages attack the buildup as an invader and begin to destroy it. This process swells and destabilizes the lesions and then they can break open and form blood clots. The more active the macrophages, the more CRP are present in the bloodstream. This type of inflammation could be categorized as subclinical or chronic inflammation that is happening at an invisible level.

Misrepair-Accumulation Theory

The misrepair-accumulation theory was suggested by Jicun Wang, Thomas M. Michelistsch, Arne Wunderlin, and Ravi Mahadeva in March 2009. This theory suggests that:

- It is the accumulation of misrepair, not the original damage, that leads to aging. Misrepair can be described as the incorrect reconstruction of a structure after repairing the original damage.[3]

For example, a cut to the skin that leaves a scar: the cut is the damage and the scar is the misrepair. The scar is considered a misrepair because the skin was not returned to its original state.

- Aging of the body occurs at the tissue level but not necessarily at the cellular and molecular level.

This theory is thought to unify the damage and programmed or genetic theories.

■ WHY ARE THESE THEORIES IMPORTANT?

Various biochemical reactions occur when we age. This leads to a significant impact on body systems. If we take a cross section of all of the proposed theories of aging, we can see that no one theory is independent of the other. They all lead to the same thing—aging.

When we age, our body systems are impacted in various ways. We cannot always see the decline, but eventually all damage will become apparent. Every aspect of our bodies will be impacted, from cells, tissues, to organs and systems. Table 4–3 depicts a chart of the aging theories and their impact on the body.

How can this information translate to the treatment room? Gaining an understanding of how the aging process may work will give the esthetician the confidence to analyze all of the treatment options available. Is it safe? Could the treatment actually work? For example, you may have an option at some point to introduce topical telomerase therapy to your clients. If you understood the telomerase theory of aging, you would know that at this time there is some risk involved for your client and that the technology is not fully developed yet. This knowledge not only protected your client but saved you a substantial capital investment.

There are so many aging theories that it is hard to determine which ones are correct and relevant to the esthetician. Even the scientists cannot agree. The following theories are widely accepted and are the ones to pay close attention to:

- Free radical theory
- Membrane theory
- Neuroendocrine theory
- Inflammation theory
- Cross linking theory
- Telomerase theory
- Mitochondrial theory

Table 4–3 Aging theories and their impact on different parts of the body.

Theory	Impact on Cells	Impact on Tissues & Organs	Impact on Body Systems
Programmed Longevity Pacemaker	Cell death or apoptosis after 50 replications Immune cells production reduced	Limited life span	Limited life span Weakened immune system
Genetic	Cell damage	Dysfunction of tissue or organs	Disease and death
Membrane	Impaired cellular communication Increased toxicity	Lipofuscin deposits increase	Disease and disorder of brain, lungs, heart, and skin
Free Radical	Impaired cellular function Metabolic waste increases to toxic levels DNA/RNA damage	Inflammation Decreased protein synthesis Organ and tissue damage	Disease and disorder of all body systems, e.g., cancer, diabetes, Alzheimer's disease, arthritis
Cross Linking	Protein binding to sugar	Thick, yellow, slack skin Cardiac impairment Renal impairment	Senile cataracts Diabetes, cancer
Mitochondrial	Reduction of ATP within cell	Organ impairment	Disease and death as organs fail
Neuroendocrine	Increased cortisol production Reduction in adequate hormones	Hypothalamus loses ability to regulate hormones Organ damage	Thyroid disease Menopause Increased body fat

Table 4–4 describes the importance of the aging theory and possible esthetic therapies that can be used to help slow the effects of aging.

Each aging theory category is responsible for multiple reactions within the body. The reality is that not one theory can stand on its own. All of these theories depend upon one another, with each system contributing. The cells may be programmed to die after a short time, which can be attributed to genetics and aggravated by free radical damage and mitochondrial impairment. Free radical damage and a high sugar diet can lead to cross linking, which will also cause stress on the neuroendocrine system. The study of aging will always be complicated and ongoing, with many different hypotheses being presented to the public. This is an area that requires constant follow-up and study for the esthetician who wants to focus on an aging clientele.

Table 4–4 A chart detailing the importance of aging theories.

Aging Theory	Why It Is Important	Possible Esthetic Therapies
Free Radical & Membrane Theory	The widely accepted expansion on the wear and tear theory. This theory will help the practitioner understand the damage that comes from environmental and lifestyle choices.	Daily antioxidant supplementation Topical application of antioxidants Professional treatment infusions of antioxidants Topical UV protection
Mitochondrial Theory	Free radical damage leads to a reduction in ATP production due to mitochondria damage, which effects how the organs function.	Daily antioxidant supplementation Topical application of antioxidants Professional treatment infusions of antioxidants Topical UV protection
Cross Linking Theory	Causes loss of elasticity.	Topical application of antioxidants Daily supplementation with essential fatty acids, reduction of simple carbohydrate intake Galvanic penetration of antioxidants Topical UV protection Increased barrier repair and restoration treatments Stress reduction techniques
Neuro-endocrine Theory	Deals with hormones and how they can affect the body.	Stress reduction techniques Massage therapy Application of topical phytoestrogens
Inflammation Theory	Long-term effects of chronic inflammation result in accumulated damage to the body.	Massage therapy Daily supplementation with essential fatty acids Low simple carbohydrate intake Stress reduction techniques Daily UV protection Professional treatment infusions of anti-oxidants and barrier repair ingredients Increased daily physical activity–especially yoga/Pilates
Telomerase Theory	Telomeres shorten each time a cell divides, which leads to cellular dysfunction, aging, and death.	Topical telomerase therapy Increased daily physical activity Stress reduction techniques Professional treatment infusions of antioxidants, retinol, and barrier repair ingredients.

■ SIGNS OF AGING

What happens to our bodies as we age is still being researched by science. New discoveries are being made all the time, but there are some well-known effects that have been quantified by science.

Each category is broken down in the same way we learn physiology in esthetic school; cells become tissues, tissues become organs, organs become systems. A simplified way of understanding the process is examining the effects of aging on the body broken down by cells, organs, and systems. All aging really starts with damage to the cell, which is the focus of most of the aging theories. This is also the area that has many scientists and doctors admitting that a good amount of information is still unproven. Listed in the sections that follow are some of the symptoms that happen to our body as we age categorized by cells, organs, and systems.

Cells

- T cells within the immune system take longer to replenish and their function is decreased.
- Body fat (adipocytes) increases generally until middle age and then starts to decrease and move internally.
- Cell division slows down and stops at around 50–60 divisions.
- Telomeres shorten, eventually leading to cell senescence.
- Reactive oxygen species (ROS) damage the cell membrane, mutate DNA, and generally cause cell injury that eventually leads to cell death.
- Cell metabolism slows down.

Organs and Body Systems

Cardiovascular:

The cardiovascular system consists of the heart, arteries, veins, blood, and red blood cells. The purpose of the system is to supply oxygen and nutrients to the body. This system is strongly affected as we age.

Heart

- Arteries stiffen and narrow with age, leading to decreased blood flow, causing our heart and other areas of the body to function at decreased levels.
- The heart pumps less efficiently. The **calcium pump protein** does not work as well.
- The heart's **ventricular walls** thicken.
- The **mitral valve** closes more slowly.
- The **SA node** loses cells. The SA node is the heart's pacemaker (pulse).

Respiratory System

The respiratory system consists of the nose, pharynx, larynx, trachea, lungs, bronchi, and alveoli. Its purpose is to provide oxygenation and excretion of carbon dioxide.

Lungs

- The capacity of the lungs decreases approximately 40 percent starting at age 20.
- The chest wall stiffens.
- The **alveoli** surface area decreases.
- Respiratory muscles weaken.

Endocrine System

The endocrine system consists of the eyes, ears, adrenals, pancreas, pineal, pituitary, thyroid, parathyroid, thymus, and gonads. These systems' purpose is to provide control and coordination, receive sensory input, transmit sensory response, regulate growth and sexual development, and maintain metabolism. This is the system that regulates hormones.

Hormones

Although not an organ or tissue, hormones have a tremendous impact on aging.

Estrogen   Estrogen slows during perimenopause and stops after menopause. Fat tissue provides smaller and weaker forms of estrogen. Skin is directly affected by the reduction of estrogen and has its own estrogen receptor.

Growth Hormone   Growth hormone is secreted by the pituitary gland to play a role in body composition and muscle and bone strength; this reduces as we age.

Testosterone   Testosterone can decline as aging progresses. Some men have no decline whereas others have. This hormone helps with sexual drive and muscle growth.

DHEA (dehydroepiandrosterone)   DHEA is produced in the adrenal glands. It is a precursor to other hormones, including testosterone and estrogen. Production peaks in the mid-20s, and gradually declines with age.

Nervous System

The nervous system controls and coordinates all other systems in the body. It consists of nerves, brain, and spinal cord.

Brain

- Connections between neurons within the brain may be reduced or seem less efficient.
- Brain cells decrease.
- Reflexes become slower.

Eyes

- Sight begins to decline starting at about 40, when seeing close detail becomes difficult.
- Eyes are less able to produce tears.
- Retinas thin and lenses become cloudy.
- Diseases and conditions such as glaucoma, macular degeneration, and cataracts increase.

Ears

- Hearing declines and the ability to hear high frequencies is reduced.
- Inner ear hair cells become damaged from sound.

Excretory System

This system consists of the kidneys, ureters, bladder and urethra, and liver. The purpose of the urinary system is water balance, formation and elimination of urine.

Kidneys

- Kidneys become less efficient at removing waste from the bloodstream.

Bladder and Urethra

- The bladder's capacity declines.
- Tissue atrophy increases with loss of estrogen, which can lead to incontinence.
- Prostrate issues can lead to incontinence.

Liver

- Liver cells become less efficient at storing and processing.

Digestive System

The gastrointestinal system consists of the mouth, esophagus, stomach, small intestine, large intestine, bile, and gallbladder. The purpose is digestion, absorption of nutrients, and elimination of waste.

Stomach

- Hydrochloric acid production declines, causing digestion to slow.
- Stomach contractions slow.
- Constipation increases.

Integumentary System

This integumenatry system consists of skin, hair and nails, sebaceous glands, and sweat glands. The purpose of this system is protection, temperature regulation, and immune response.

Skin

The skin shows multiple age-related issues such as the following:

- Dry skin increases.
- The signs of photodamage become more apparent, such as hypo-/hyperpigmentation, texture roughness, precancerous lesions, and increased bruising.
- Thinning of the dermis—reduced as much as 20 percent in elderly patients.[4]
- Decreased desquamation (cell turnover). Rate slows from 30 percent to 50 percent between ages 30 and 80.[5]
- Reduced ability to repair damage.
- Loss of temperature control.
- Reduced immune response.
- Collagen content per unit area of skin surface decreases at 1 percent per year as we age, and dermis develops fragmented elastic fibers. Type I collagen decreases, Type III collagen increases.[6]
- Elastin structure changes and GAG's within the dermis may decrease, leading to wrinkling, diminished capacity to support the microcirculation, and decreased skin strength.
- Increased instance of disorders, for example rosacea.
- Venous structure decreases by 35 percent compared to young skin.[7]
- Sebaceous glands become larger and sebum production decreases.[8]
- Melanocytes number decreases 8 percent to 20 percent per decade, which leads to increased cancer risk.[9]

Skeletal System

Consists of bones, joints, cartilage. This system is responsible for support and protection, and red blood cell production.

- Bone mass and size decreases.
- Joints can become inflamed and stiff.

Lymphatic System

This system includes the white blood cells, lymph vessels and nodes, spleen, tonsils, and appendix. It is responsible for protection and repair of the body.

- Increases in pro-inflammatory cytokines.

- Body is less able to fight infections.
- Lymph circulation slows.

Muscular System

This system includes muscles and tendons. It is responsible for body movement and internal fluid circulation.

- Muscle mass declines and strength is reduced.
- Flexibility is reduced.

▶ ❯ ❯ Top Ten Tips to Take to the Clinic

1. The cause of aging is unknown at this time.
2. Only one theory has been proven conclusively.
3. Aging is inevitable and cannot be stopped.
4. Slowing the aging process is possible.
5. Collagen decreases by 1 percent per year.
6. Intrinsic aging refers to the effects of genetics.
7. Extrinsic aging refers to lifestyle choices.
8. Damage control theories relate to the damage done by lifestyle choices.
9. Programmed theories relate to genetics.
10. Inflammation theory should be understood by the esthetician, because many treatments are performed to promote the wound-healing process.

Chapter Review Questions

1. What are the most widely accepted aging theories?
2. What is the term *senescence* related to?
3. What is macro aging?
4. What is micro aging?
5. What is the telomerase theory of aging?
6. What is the inflammation theory of aging?

References

1. Funk, W. D., Wang, C. K., Shelton, D. N., Harley, C. B., Pagon G. D., Hoeffler, W. K. (2000). "Telomerase Expression Restores Dermal Integrity to In Vitro-aged Fibroblasts in a Reconstituted Skin Model." *Experimental Cell Research*, Volume 258, Issue 2, 270–278.
2. Pugliese, P. MD. (2001). *Physiology of the Skin II*. Carol Stream, IL: Allured Publishing.
3. Wang, J., Michelitsch, T., Wunderlin, A., Mahadeva, R. (2009). *Aging as a Consequence of Misrepair—A Novel Theory of Aging*. Nature Precedings, *arXiv:0904.0575*. http://arxiv.org/abs/0904.0575.
4. Baumann, L. MD., Saghari, S. MD., Weisburg, E. MS., (2009). *Cosmetic Dermatology: Principles and Practice*, 2nd Edition. New York, NY: Mc Graw Hill Medical.
5. Baumann, L. MD., Saghari, S. MD., Weisburg, E. MS., (2009). *Cosmetic Dermatology: Principles and Practice*, 2nd Edition. New York, NY: Mc Graw Hill Medical.
6. Baumann, L. MD., Saghari, S. MD., Weisburg, E. MS., (2009). *Cosmetic Dermatology: Principles and Practice*, 2nd Edition. New York, NY: Mc Graw Hill Medical.
7. Baumann, L. MD., Saghari, S. MD., Weisburg, E. MS., (2009). *Cosmetic Dermatology: Principles and Practice*, 2nd Edition. New York, NY: Mc Graw Hill Medical.
8. Baumann, L. MD., Saghari, S. MD., Weisburg, E. MS., (2009). *Cosmetic Dermatology: Principles and Practice*, 2nd Edition. New York, NY: Mc Graw Hill Medical.
9. Baumann, L. MD., Saghari, S. MD., Weisburg, E. MS., (2009). *Cosmetic Dermatology: Principles and Practice*, 2nd Edition. New York, NY: Mc Graw Hill Medical.

Bibliography

Colbert, B., Ankey, J., Wilson, J., Havrilla, J. (1997). *An Integrated Approach to Health Sciences: Anatomy and Physiology, Math, Physics, and Chemistry*. New York: Delmar Publishers.

de Magalhães, J. P., Toussaint, O. (July 2004). "Telomeres and Telomerase: A Modern Fountain of Youth?" *Rejuvenation Research*, 7(2): 126–133.

Gowan, K. (2009). "Can We Cure Aging? The New Science of Health." *Discover Magazine*, Summer: 5–8.

Harman, D. (1992). "Role of Free Radicals in Aging and Disease." *Annals of New York Academy of Sciences*, 2:332–3.

Masoro, E. J., Austad, S. N. (2006). *Handbook of the Biology of Aging,* Sixth Edition. San Diego: Academic Press.

Moody, H. (2006). *Aging: Concepts and Controversies*, 5th Edition. Thousand Oaks, CA: Pine Forge Press.

Pugliese, P. MD. (2005). *Advanced Professional Skin Care*, Medical Edition. Bernville, PA: The Topical Agent LLC.

Perricone, P. MD. (2000). *The Wrinkle Cure: Unlock the Power of Cosmeceuticals for Supple, Youthful Skin*. New York: Warner Books.

Rizzo, D. PHD. (2007). *Fundamentals of Anatomy and Physiology*, 2nd Edition. Clifton Park, NY: Delmar Cengage Learning.

Szilard, L. (1958). On the Nature of the Aging Process. University of Chicago UP, department of genetics paper N. 712.

Zs-Nagy, I. (1992). "A Proposal for Reconsideration of the Role of Oxygen Free Radicals in Cell Differentiation and Aging." *Annals of the New York Academy of Sciences*, 1992, 673: 142–8.

Website

www.nia.nih.gov

The Healthy Aging Skin Treatment Program

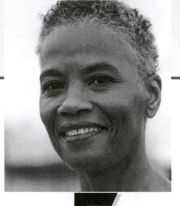

Chapter 5

Key Terms

7-dehydrocholesterol
fatty acid
acid mantle
corneocytes
corynebacterium
dynamic expression
lines
eledin
epidermal lipids
fascia
filaggrin
free sterols
glycoproteins
keratosis pilaris
lamellar bodies
natural moisture
factors (NMF)
odland bodies
Propionobacterium
(P. Acnes)
RETE ridges
sphingolipids
Staphylococcus
aureus
Staphylococcus
epidermidis

keratohyaline granules
profilaggrin
transglutaminases
(Tgase)
lamellar bodies
desmosomes
ceramide
cholesterol
melanocytes
aquaporin channels
epidermal growth
factor (EGF)
epidermal growth
factor receptor
(EGFR)
tyrosine kinase
activity
keratinocyte growth
factor (KGF)
polypeptide growth
factors
TGF-a
TGF-b
extracellular matrix
(ECM)
fibroblasts

fibrocytes
fibrillin
fibronectin
lamin
glycosaminoglycans
keratinization
essential fatty acid
deficiency (EFAD)
elastase
collagenase (MMPs)
AP-1
inflammatory
cytokines
proteasome enzyme
complex
ER-B
ER-A
Advanced glycation
end products
(AGEs)
permanent elastotic
creases
static rhytids
atrophic crinkling
rhytids
gravitational fold

ACTH (adrenocorticotropic) stress hormone
POMC (proopiomelanocortin)
MSH (melanin stimulating hormone)

melanocortin
tyrosinase
melanosome
transepidermal water loss (TEWL)
transient amplifying (TA) cells

TIMPs
mast cells
proteoglycans

Learning Objectives

After completing this chapter, you will be able to:

1. Understand the structure and function of the skin.

2. Identify how to assess aging skin conditions.

3. Identify solutions to treat aging skin conditions.

4. Learn how to put a complete esthetic treatment plan together.

Why Is This Important?

Understanding the biological function of each layer of skin is vitally important to determine if the products you are using are correct and if the chosen treatments can actually impact the skin. If you don't understand HOW the product/treatment works, how can you know WHY you should use it and be able to explain it to your client.

tran epidermal water loss (TEWL)

The process that allows epidermal water loss; impacted by an impaired acid mantle.

acid mantle

skin layer that is a complex fluid at a pH of 4.5 to 5.5 formed by the excretions from sebaceous, sodiferious glands, epidermal lipids, and NMF (natural moisture factor); contains 7 dehydrocholesterol fatty acid. This layer has *micro flora* that contribute to the skin's first layer barrier defense.

epidermal lipids

important part of the structure of the epidermis; prevents TEWL. Includes triglycerides, fatty acids, squalene, wax esters, and cholesterol; can be affected by diet, genetics, environment and aging.

7-dehydrocholestrol fatty acid

fatty acid that provides the body with vitamin d3 through the conversion of ultraviolet light.

▪ CREATING A COMPREHENSIVE PLAN FOR YOUR CLIENT

Creating a comprehensive plan for our client is one of the most challenging and satisfying parts of treating an aging client. This portion of the consultation process is always a challenge but can be very rewarding. It also is very flexible, as a comprehensive plan should be evaluated at each client visit. Understanding all modalities offered to the client and the basic physiology of the skin is an important part of creating a treatment plan that will give the client effective results. This chapter will give you an outline of the basic conditions of an aging skin and solutions available.

▪ CHALLENGES AND SOLUTIONS

Understanding the skin is the core of knowledge the esthetician needs and there are many resources available for the esthetician to increase knowledge. It is helpful when treating aging skin to be able to link the structure and function of the skin to the condition that needs to be treated. For example, dehydration is one of the most common conditions seen in aging skin, but it is more than just increased **transepidermal water loss** (**TEWL**). What is really causing it? This is where understanding the desquamation process and the enzymes involved is very valuable. Let's look at the structure and functions of the skin in this simple manner. You will also find a fold-out illustration detailing the skin layers and functions within the insert of this text.

▪ SKIN LAYERS OF THE EPIDERMIS

The skin has six layers within the epidermis including the addition of the **acid mantle**, and each layer has a role to play. They are:

Acid Mantle

Structure: This layer is actually a complex fluid formed by the excretions from sebaceous, sudoriferous glands, **epidermal lipids**, and NMF (natural moisture factor) and contains **7-dehydrocholesterol fatty acid**. This layer has "micro flora" that contributes to the skins first layer barrier defense. The micro flora in the acid mantle known at this time are:

- **Staphylococcus aureus**
- **Staphylococcus epidermidis**
- **Propionobacterium (P. Acnes)** — this bacteria helps with the creation of free fatty acids which are responsible for the acid pH of the acid mantle; it is also a factor in acne.[1]
- **Corynebacterium**
- Various Gram-negative bacteria

Function: maintain pH of 5.5 on the skin, inhibit growth of harmful bacteria, prevent *TEWL* (transepidermal water loss), prevent toxins from being absorbed into skin, promote the creation of vitamin D through UV exposure on 7-dehydrocholesterol fatty acid, and act as a lubricant on surface of skin.

Stratum Corneum

Structure: also known as the horny layer, it consists of **corneocytes**, which are cells without a nucleus and cellular structure; they are filled with keratin proteins, with lipids surrounding them in the extracellular space. The cells are connected to each other by corneodesmosomes, which are protein bridges that look similar to small hair-like projections. This layer is often described with the "brick and mortar" analogy, referring to the corneocytes as the bricks and the lipids that surround the cell as mortar (Figure 5–1). Within this intercellular space are lamellar bodies.

    Function: its primary role is protection and generation of **natural moisturizing factors** (**NMF**) in the skin. It regulates moisture balance, and is 15 cell layers thick.[2] NMF is created by enzymes breaking down the keratin-filaggrin complex to separate **filaggrin** and keratin, and then proteolytic enzymes are further activated when the water content in the stratum corneum is decreased. This breaks down filaggrin into amino acids that help form NMF, which is the natural physical barrier of the skin and helps rehydrate the skin. **Lamellar bodies** secrete **free sterols**, **sphingolipids**, and **glycoproteins**, which allow a balance of both hydrophilic and lipophilic materials to pass through the stratum corneum.[3] Cells in this layer are dead, with no nucleus or organelles.

Stratum Lucidum

Structure: a clear cellular layer, filled with **eledin**, which is the precursor molecule to keratin.

    Function: continued formation of the bilayers through the secretion of **odland bodies**, and the keratinization process continues with

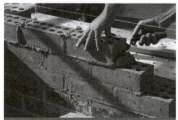

© John Leung, 2010. Used under license from shutterstock.com.

Figure 5–1 The stratum corneum layer is often described with the "brick and mortar" analogy, referring to the corneocytes as the bricks and the lipids that surround the cell as mortar.

keratohyalin creating eledin, which in turn forms keratin. Cells in this layer are dead, having no nucleus and organelles.

Stratum Granulosom

Structure: granular layer consists of **keratohyaline granules** containing **profilaggrin** and cornified cell proteins cross linked by the calcium requiring enzymes **transglutaminases** (TGase).[4] Organelles called **lamellar bodies**, which are key for the production of barrier lipids, are also present. Connecting the keratinocytes, which have become granular and less flexible, are the **desmosomes**, which are hair-like appendages that hold cells together in order to maintain correct continual cell maturation and differentiation. Cells are beginning to die.

   Function: responsible for formation of amino acids that create NMF and dissolving of the desmosomes.

Stratum Spinosum

Structure: spiny layer, the thickest layer, keratinization process begins here. Cells have nucleus and organelles and are considered alive. This layer also has the densest concentration of hyaluronic acid.[5]

   Function: this layer is very important to the immune system. Cellular changes such as the formation of odland bodies, which is a granule that contains **ceramide**, **cholesterol**, and free fatty acids, start here. **Melanocytes** synthesize melanin and transfer melansome granules via microtubes to keratinocytes. **Aquaporin channels** are thought to impact keratinocytes by facilitating transport of water, glycerol, and solutes.[6]

Stratum Basale (Germinativum) and Dermal/Epidermal Junction

Structure: basal cell layer is also known as the basement membrane, it connects to the spiny layer through the desmosomes and the dermis by the **RETE ridges**. Keratinocyte stem cells located at RETE ridges create **transient amplifying (TA) cells**, which divide. Ten percent (10%) of the basale cells are stem cells, fifty percent (50%) are amplifying cells, and forty percent (40%) are post-mitotic cells.[7] Keratinocytes surround the melanocytes, Langerhans, and Merkel cells connected by

The difference in skin color is due to the size and distribution of the melanocytes, as well as the amount of melanin produced. We are all born with the same number of melanocytes. A new approach in treating skin of color is to look at the individual's healing response time instead of genetic makeup (hair, eye color, etc.).

Stem cells are slowly dividing cells which proliferate less often as the body ages or is exposed to environmental damage. In skin, they are found in the RETE ridges and the outer root sheath of the hair follicle. These cells can replicate themselves or turn into different cell types. Certain conditions such as wound healing or exposure to growth factors can influence stem cells to divide faster. A foreign stem cell, such as one from a plant, cannot replace a human stem cell. It is possible to stimulate stem cell activity through controlled wounding, and possibly some cosmeceutical ingredients.

hemi-desmosomes. Aquaporin channels are thought to impact keratino-cytes as well.

Function: responsible for maintaining the epidermis by continually renewing, RETE pegs connect the epidermis to dermis, melanocytes are found here, TA cells are responsible for the most cell division.[8] Growth factors such as **epidermal growth factor (EGF)** bind to the **epidermal growth factor receptor (EGFR)** and activate **tyrosine kinase activity**, which results in cell proliferation. Also present is **keratinocyte growth factor (KGF),** which enhances hyaluronan synthesis, cell proliferation, and wound healing. Also present in the basal layer are **polypeptide growth factors TGF-a and TGF-b.** TGF-a is similar to EGF in that it stimulates the tyrosine kinase activity, and TGF-b promotes cell differentiation and is shown to have role in scarring. Located also in the basement membrane are **proteoglycans** and collagen types IV and VII.[9]

The dermis is where the primary aging of the skin takes place. Changing the structure and function of the dermis is out of the scope of practice for an esthetician, but there are therapies that indirectly affect the dermis in many ways. Loss of firmness is an example of one of the most obvious effects of an aging dermis, and one of the hardest to address as well. Understanding how the dermis works will help you design an effective plan of treatment.

■ SKIN LAYERS OF THE DERMIS

The dermis has three layers each working together to support the epidermis. They are:

Papillary Layer

Structure: most active layer, and is made up of loose collagen and elastin fibers known as areolar surrounded by glycosaminoglycans (GAGs) as well as **mast cells**, phagocytes, white blood cells, fibroblasts, and fibrocytes. Blood, lymph vessels, sebaceous, sudoriferous glands, and shafts of hair follicles are also are found here. At the top of the papillary layer is the dermal/epidermal junction.

Function: to provide support and strength to the skin.

---

fillagrin
filament aggregating protein; binds keratin filaments to form a structural matrix in the stratum corneum; the breakdown of filaggrin contributes to NMF (natural moisturizing factor).

lamellar bodies
formed in the keratinocytes of the stratum spinosum and stratum granulosum. When the keratinocyte matures to the stratum corneum, enzymes degrade the outer envelope of the lamellar bodies releasing types of lipids called free fatty acids and ceramides.

free sterols
group of natural steroid alcohols, such as cholesterol and ergosterol, which are waxy insoluble substances.

sphingolipids
ipids derived from sphingosine; important for cell functions.

glycoproteins
any of a group of conjugated proteins having a carbohydrate as the nonprotein component; important membrane proteins, which play a role in cell to cell interactions.

eledin
presursor molecule to the formation of keratin.

odland bodies
secretory organelles found in stratum granulosum layer of the epidermis; lamellar bodies are released from keratinocytes into the intercellular spaces to form an impermeable, lipid-containing sheet that serves to form a water barrier.

keratohyline granules
any of the irregularly shaped granules present in the cells of the granular layer of the epidermis.

profillaggrin
a structural protein synthesized by cells of the stratum granulosum and a precursor of filaggrin.

transglutaminases (Tgase)
involved in the formation of the cornified cell envelope by cross-linking a variety of structural proteins in the epidermis.

lamellar bodies
formed in the keratinocytes of the stratum spinosum and stratum granulosum. When the keratinocyte matures to the stratum corneum, enzymes degrade the outer envelope of the lamellar bodies releasing types of lipids called free fatty acids and ceramides.

desmosomes
small hair-like protrusions that hold cells together; integral for cell transport.

Reticular Layer

Structure: located below the papillary layer, has dense type III collagen and elastin, giving the skin its strength and structure. In this layer as well as the papillary layer is the **extracellular matrix (ECM)** or ground substance. Within the ground substance are **fibroblasts, fibrocytes, fibrillin, fibronectin,** and **lamin** as well as **glycosaminoglycans**.

Function: ground substance surrounds all the cells of the dermis and gives shape and structure to the dermis. The reticular layer is important for cell-to-cell signaling, wound repair, cell adhesion, positioning, proliferation, identity, and fate. Fibroblasts are responsible for creating the ground substance as well as maintaining it.

Subcutaneous Layer

Structure: this layer is also known as subcutis and is made up of fat cells, blood vessels, lymph vessels, nerve fibers, and loose connective tissue. The base of hair follicles and sweat glands can protrude into this layer.

Function: to give shape and strength to the skin, temperature regulation, and mechanical protection.

CONDITION: HYPERKERATINIZATION (DEAD SKIN CELL BUILDUP)

Hyperkeratinization or dead skin cell buildup is a very common condition that affects the texture of the skin. Any skin type can have it and it is not necessarily only an aging skin problem, but will make fine lines and wrinkles seem worse than they are (Figure 5–2).

The first visual signs that you may see within the client's skin are:

- Fine surface wrinkles
- Dehydration—parchment paper look
- Comedones/milia
- Dull skin
- Grayish color tone

Figure 5–2 Hyperkeratinization or dead skin buildup as it affects the skin.

- Flakey skin
- Light reflective sheen

Cause of Hyperkeratinization

This condition can be correlated with several processes within the skin. They are a malfunction in the **keratinization** process in which desmosomes are not dissolving efficiently. Desmosomes are the hair-like protrusions on the epithelial cell that hold them together. Increased transepidermal water loss (TEWL) lowers the natural moisturizing factor (NMF) of the skin, and this impairs the amount of water available within the skin and the ability of epidermal enzymes to function correctly. Also impacting the desquamation of the skin is **essential fatty acid deficiency** (**EFAD**), which results in poor alignment of bilayers and sticky corneocytes.

The texture of the skin is the first place to show the signs of aging. When looking at the texture of the skin it is important to understand the structure and function of the epidermis as well as the dermis. The cell renewal process as well as desquamation is important to the texture of the skin and when either of these processes is abnormal it directly affects the visual appearance as well as the immune function of the skin.

Diagnostic Signs

- Skin looks uneven, with a light reflective sheen.
- Skin feels rough and possibly looks flakey.
- When pressure is applied in an upward direction, the skin will have a crêpe or parchment paper look.
- Eye area shows signs of fine lines and crinkly appearance.
- Woods lamp will show a white fluorescence throughout the face.
- Fine surface lines in a cross hatch or linear pattern are apparent without touch.
- **Keratosis pilaris** may be present on the body.

Solutions

Esthetic Treatments

Goal: Increase cell turnover rate by breaking desmosomes and stimulating cellular function through increasing free water in epidermis to support optimal enzyme function.

---

ceramide
a molecule within the lipid family, made of a sphingosine plus a fatty acid, naturally found within the skin.

cholesterol
thick lipid molecule found within cell membranes and transported within blood plasma; needed for healthy cell function.

melanocytes
melanin-producing cells located in the stratum basale.

aquaporin channels
water channels that transport water across cell membranes made of specialized membrane proteins known as aquaporins. Discovered by Peter Agre who jointly won a Nobel Prize in 2003.

RETE ridges
epidermal thickenings that extend downward between dermal papillae

TA (transient amplifying) cells
cells that are involved in differentiation also called daughter cells.

epidermal growth factor (EGF)
a protein molecule or steroid hormone that stimulates proliferation and differentiation of epidermal cells.

epidermal growth factor receptor (EGFR)
a receptor found in epidermal cells that enables EGF to function.

tyrosine kinase activity
A group of enzymes important in cell growth, differentiation, and development.

keratinocyte growth factor (KGF)
a growth factor present in the epithelialization-phase of wound healing. In this phase, keratinocytes are covering the wound, forming the epithelium.

polypeptide growth factors
protein that controls proliferation, cellular differentiation, and other functions in most cells.

TGF-a
protein that controls proliferation, cellular differentiation, and other functions in most cells.

TGF-b
protein that controls proliferation, cellular differentiation, and other functions in most cells.

protoeoglycans
a glycoprotein which is a major component of the extracellular matrix

mast cells
play a central role in inflammatory and immediate allergic reactions, found in tissues throughout the body, particularly in association with structures such as blood vessels and nerves.

extracellular matrix (ECM)
a network of non-living tissues which provides support, regulates communication, and encourages growth, healing, and adhesion for cells. Skin has a large extracellular matrix which keeps the skin strong and young looking.

fibroblasts
cell in connective tissue that synthesizes collagen.

Options:
- Chemical Peeling: AHAs, Enzymes
- Mechanical Exfoliation: Microdermabrasion, Scrubs, Ultrasonic
- Facial Treatments: Focus on hydration of skin (hyaluronic acid, ceramides, and essential fatty acids), mild exfoliation, stimulating massage (unless sensitivity is present), lymphatic drainage massage, and iontophoresis (galvanic current).

Medical Treatments

Goal: Remove layers of the stratum corneum by chemical or physical means.

- Medical Chemical Peels
- Laser Treatments
- Prescriptions: Tretinoin—Retin-A, Ammonium Lactate—Lac-Hydrin

Professional Products:

Sun protection is mandatory for all skin conditions.

Cleansers/Toners: Use neutral pH cleansers with limited surfactants, glycolic cleansers or enzymes. Non-alcohol-based toners.

Treatment Products and Moisturizers: Use the following ingredients:

- Serums with hyaluronic acid
- Ceramides
- Free fatty acids
- Lactic acid
- Glycolic acid
- Salicylic acid (if genetic skin type is oily)
- Retinol or retinaldehyde
- Essential fatty acids

Lifestyle Choices

Basic healthy lifestyle choices such as:

- Increased daily aerobic fitness
- Daily sun protection
- Diet consisting of a balance of vegetables, fruits, proteins, and adequate water

CONDITION: DEHYDRATION (FAST TEWL)

Dehydration is the most common condition that the esthetician deals with. Many products are focused on dealing with this issue. With an aging skin this is not the primary condition to treat but will impact how the skin looks and functions. Any genetic skin type can have this condition. The first visual signs (Figure 5–3) that you may see within the client's skin are:

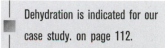

Dehydration is indicated for our case study. on page 112.

- Surface wrinkles
- Lines at sides of eye (smile lines)
- Dull rough skin
- Gray to yellow pallor
- Flakey skin
- Possible redness through cheek area and nose

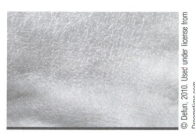

© Defun, 2010. Used under license from Dreamstime.com.

Figure 5–3 Dehydrated skin is a common condition that estheticians deal with.

Cause of Dehydration

Dehydration has a large lifestyle component that the esthetician needs to take into account. Caffeine, water, and medication intake is vitally important. Low ambient humidity has an impact on how the skin regulates TEWL. When extracellular and intracellular fluids are imbalanced, this leads to less free water within the epidermis, which impairs enzyme activity. This affects the digestion process of filaggrin starting in the granular layer, which directly affects the NMF of the epidermis and the processing of amino acids. An impaired acid mantle also has an important role in slowing TEWL and retaining water. This should also be a focus in treatment.

The GAGs of the dermis are where the lack of water begins and is directly affected by poor microcirculation, including poor lymphatic circulation. Capillaries (lymph and blood) release water, nutrients, proteins, and oxygen into the extracellular space in the dermis, feeding the cells. This fluid rises up through the dermal/epidermal junction to the basal layer, impacting the regeneration of new cells. If the dermis is impacted, which is very dependent on lifestyle habits, the skin will have a very hard time retaining a good moisture balance.

fibrocyte
long spindle shaped cells found along bundles of collagen that are the principle cells of connective tissue, they help maintain the ground substance of the dermis.

fibrillin
small fibers that are a component of elastin.

fibronection
a cell adhesion molecule that anchors cells to collagen or proteoglycans.

lamin
fibrous proteins providing structural function and communication regulation within the cell.

glycosaminoglycans
GAGs form an important component of connective tissues.

keratinization
process in which desmosomes are not dissolving efficiently which causes a dead skin cell build up.

desmosomes
small hair-like protrusions that hold cells together; integral for cell transport.

essential fatty acid deficiency (EFAD)
lack of essential fatty acids such as omegas 3 and 6. The body cannot manufacture essential fatty acids as they must be ingested.

keratosis pilaris
genetic follicular condition that appears as red raised bumps on the skin.

Diagnostic Signs

- Dry scratchy skin
- Puffy eyes (impaired lymphatic drainage system)
- Easily irritated skin
- Diffused redness (rosacea)
- Hyperkeratinized skin
- Possible stinging and tightness after cleansing
- Woods lamp will show a light purple fluorescence throughout the face
- Damage to the skin is slow to heal
- Fine lining present (parchment paper look) when skin is touched
- Client could have high caffeine intake, low water intake, essential fatty acid deficiency, and work/live in low ambient humidity

Solutions

Esthetic Treatments

Goal: Increase the amount of free water and lipids with in skin, slow TEWL, and improve microcirculation, including lymph circulation.

Options:
- Chemical Peeling: Lactic acid
- Facial Treatments: Focus on hydration of skin (hyaluronic acid, ceramides, and essential fatty acids), mild enzyme exfoliation, lymphatic drainage massage, and penetration of hydrating serums with iontophoresis (galvanic current) or LLT sonophoresis.

Medical Treatments

Goal: This condition is not usually the primary concern within a medical setting.

Professional Products

Cleansers/Toners: Focus on gentle, nonsurfactant, neutral pH cleanser.

Treatment Products and Moisturizers: Use the following ingredients:

- Ceramides
- Essential fatty acids
- Sphingolipids
- Cholesterol
- Silicones

- Algae
- Hyaluronic acid
- Calcium
- Niacinamide

Lifestyle Choices

Dehydration is the one condition that is directly related to the client's lifestyle choices. The following lifestyle choices need to be addressed:

- Daily intake of water; adequate levels are needed based on body weight and lifestyle.
- Daily intake of caffeine or other diuretics, including alcohol.
- Essential fatty acid deficiency, usually from low-fat diet or chronic dieting.
- Smoking.
- Prescription medication, including over-the-counter sinus/cold/allergy medication.
- Amount of time spent in low ambient humidity (air conditioning, central heat, etc.).
- Daily fitness levels (this will improve microcirculation).

AGING SKIN CONDITIONS

Cause

Aging is a complicated process that involves multiple biologic reactions. These processes are different in each person and one common cause is not known due to the client's genetic makeup and lifestyle choices. The study of aging is ongoing, with new theories and studies released often. It is a good idea for the esthetician to understand these possible causes in order create an effective program. The general process of aging skin will be outlined in this section then divided into stages to give general guidelines on treatment. Each stage of aging will have close to the same challenges, but with each stage the intensity is increased.

There are three influencing factors to consider when looking at the process of aging skin. They are:

UV Radiation Exposure

UV exposure affects the skin by increasing the production of **elastase** and **collagenase** (MMPs) through the activation of **AP-1**, inactivating

elastase
the enzyme that activates elastosis.

collagenase
an enzyme that controls the removal of collagen with in the body.

AP-1
transcription factor which regulates gene expression and controls cellular processes in response to a variety of stimuli, including cytokines, growth factors, stress, and bacterial and viral infections

Aging is often referred to as extrinsic and intrinsic. Intrinsic aging is theorized to be related to genetics or DNA replication issues (Hayflick theory). Extrinsic is directly related to lifestyle, with UV radiation exposure the primary factor and the cause of many of the listed processes.

> The body cannot repair damaged proteins, only remove them. When that process is impaired, all cellular processes can become impaired.

> The skin cannot absorb oxygen from the outside in; spraying oxygen on the stratum corneum does not cause the skin to absorb oxygen. That happens with a complex biological process that begins with the circulatory system and requires iron. Iron is required to transport oxygen and is also a cofactor in the synthesis of collagen.

> Free water content is impacted by the lymphatic system, medications, and water intake.

inflammatory cytokines
any of a number of small proteins that are secreted by specific cells of the immune system which carry signals locally between cells, to increase inflammation in response to immune system activation.

proteosome enzyme complex
a protein group found with in the cells; degrades and digests damaged proteins through proteolysis.

vitamin A receptors, increasing the formation of free radicals which cause perioxidation of cellular lipids, vitamin C oxidation, activation of melanosomes, and **inflammatory cytokines**.

Skin Health

The effects of aging directly relate to levels of hydration in the skin, which are essential for enzyme function and essential fatty acid deficiency, which is essential for the creation of prostaglandins.[10] This affects aging skin by lowering the amount of TIMPs available to regulate MMPs and the health of the phospholipids in the cell wall. Lower TIMPs lead to reduced proteolysis (proteosomal decline), which is an essential enzyme function that removes damaged proteins within the body. This process is regulated by **proteasome enzyme complex** and affects all cellular processes.

Chronic subclinical inflammation also contributes to this process by increasing proinflammatory cytokines, which help degrade collagen and elastin. Hormonal changes also disrupt skin health. There are three hormone receptors found in skin cells: an androgen receptor and two estrogen receptors, **ER-B** and **ER-A**. ER-B is localized in the fibroblasts of the dermis, which are responsible for the synthesis of collagen, elastin, and the ECM (extracellular matrix) or ground substance.

Oxygen absorption loss is another factor in the aging process. After age 70 the cells, ability to absorb oxygen decreases 30 percent, Lifestyle choices also impact the cells, ability to absorb oxygen. This leads to slow stem cell differentiation, slows desquamation, and impairs the fibroblasts, ability to produce GAGs, collagen, and elastin.

Advanced glycation end products (AGEs) are also related to skin health. The process of glycation binds a sugar molecule to protein, which creates oxidative stress and increases inflammatory cytokines. If the proteasome enzyme complex is impaired, damage will accelerate.

Genetics

Genetics affect skin aging by processes that are out of our control at this point in science. With age comes a natural reduction in TIMPs, growth factors, and hormones. Telomeres also play an important role (see Chapter 4, Basics of Aging). These telomeres shorten every time the cell replicates, eventually leading to cell senescence.

All of these influencing factors lead directly to cellular processes being impaired that are necessary for differentiation, signaling, metabolism, and

DNA repair. Impaired cellular processes will directly affect the fibroblasts, ability to create collagen, elastin, and GAGs, which impacts the structure of the dermis.

Reduced fascia strength is the result of the structure of the superficial and deep fascia being impacted by impaired cellular processes, all influenced by the proceeding factors. Also involved are the muscles. Muscles play a part in the process by pulling down on the fiber matrix of the skin, which includes collagen and elastin. Wrinkles form across muscle in an up-and-down or perpendicular pattern (Figure 5–4).

When the skin loses collagen and elastin, it cannot stay firm, and a wrinkle will develop. The muscles of the face are attached to the skin via **fascia** where the collagen and elastin are. When these become weak, they are no longer able to resist the pull of gravity or muscle contraction. When muscle contraction is lessened or stopped, as with the use of Botox®, the skin will not form deep wrinkles.

ER-B

a estrogen receptor found on skin cells. 2nd type found.

ER-A

androgen receptor and estrogen receptor found on skin cells.

Advanced Glycation End Products (AGE's)

process of glycation; binds a sugar molecule to protein which creates oxidative stress, and increases inflammatory cytokines

fascia

a sheet or band of fibrous connective tissue enveloping, separating, or binding together muscles, organs, and other soft structures of the body.

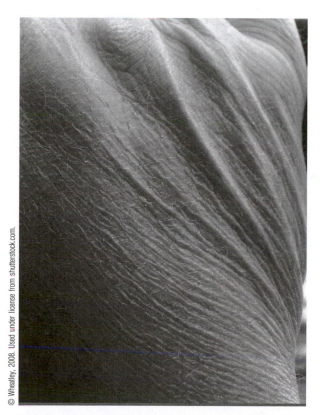

© Wheatley, 2008. Used under license from shutterstock.com.

Figure 5–4 Wrinkles develop when the skin loses collagen and elastin.

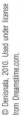

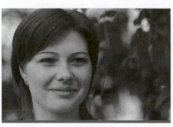

Figure 5–5 Stage 1: Fine wrinkles are often the first signs of aging.

This stage of aging reflects the conditions seen in the objective analysis of our case study on page 112.

dynamic expression lines
aging lines that are more apparent with facial movement.

CONDITION: STAGE 1: FINE WRINKLES—MILD ELASTOSIS—MILD PHOTODAMAGE

The first visual signs that you may see (Figure 5–5) within the client's skin are:

- Lines at sides of eye and upper lip with facial movement
- Mild hyperpigmentation
- Mild nasolabial fold depth
- Fine visible capillaries
- Rough texture, increased fine wrinkles, and dark circles around eyes

Diagnostic Signs

- Fine texture changes—general roughness
- Fine lines visible with facial movement
- **Dynamic expression lines**: These are the typical frown lines, laugh lines, and crows' feet. These wrinkles respond well to Botox®, as shown in Figure 5–6.
- Mild hyperpigmentation or general dull appearance to skin
- Nasolabial fold beginning to become pronounced
- Mild skin fold at edge of ear when laying down
- Photodamage apparent under Woods lamp—deep dermal layer (light brown) spots and epidermal layer (dark brown), elastosis will show around eyes with a purple color
- Increased dryness or dehydration in skin due to hormonal changes; shows as light purple under Woods lamp
- Increased redness or sensitivity
- Small vertical lines found at tear ducts and or lash line and rough texture around eyes
- Small vertical lines on upper lip area

Solutions

Esthetic Treatments

Goal: Prevent further UV radiation damage, reduce lipid peroxidation, increase antioxidant protection, increase microcirculation and lymphatic flow (oxygen transport), reduce TEWL, increase fibroblast stimulation, stimulate stem cell proliferation, reduce glycation, slow MMP activation, and reduce chronic inflammation.

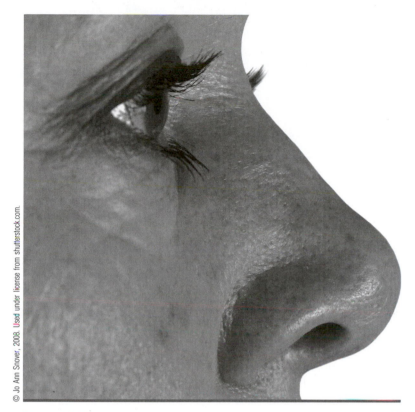

Figure 5–6 Dynamic expression lines are typical frown lines, laugh lines, and crows' feet.

Options:

- Chemical Peeling: Lactic Acid, Glycolic Acid, Enzymes, Modified Jessneral's, Mild TCA (>7%)
- Mechanical Exfoliation: Microdermabrasion, Ultrasonic
- Facial Treatments: Focus on antioxidant infusion and hydration (hyaluronic acid, ceramides, algae, and essential fatty acids), mild exfoliation, lymphatic drainage massage, firming compression masks, and iontophoresis (galvanic current). Low-level sonophoresis, microcurrent, LED light therapy.

Medical Treatments

Goal: Stimulate production of collagen, inhibit melanosomes, relax wrinkles, and prevent UV damage.

Treatments:

- IPL/photopneumatic
- Fractionated lasers

- Radiofrequency and infrared skin tightening
- Botox
- Retinoids
- Superficial peels
- Hydroquinone

Professional Products

Sunscreen daily is mandatory to prevent further damage.

Cleansers/Toners: Appropriate for skin type, possibly with a mild AHA or enzyme. Tonic with peptides or focusing on increasing water content in stratum corneum.

Treatment Products and Moisturizers: Look for some of the following ingredients:

- Ceramides
- Essential fatty acids
- Sphingolipids
- Silicones
- Algae
- Hyaluronic acid
- Calcium
- Niacinamide
- Retinaldehyde/Retinol
- Peptides: wrinkle smoothing, pigment inhibitors, antioxidant
- Magnesium ascorbyl phosphate
- Antioxidants: ALL
- Soy
- Pycnogenol
- Beta glucan
- Arbutin
- Malus domestica (Phyto Cell Tech)
- Phycosaccharide Al (Phycojuvenine)
- Paper mulberry

Lifestyle Choices

Stage 1 aging is affected directly by lifestyle choices. The following lifestyle choices need to be addressed:

- Daily intake of water; adequate levels are needed based on body weight and lifestyle.
- Daily UV radiation protection.

- Essential fatty acid deficiency, usually from low-fat diet or chronic dieting.
- Smoking, alcohol intake.
- Diet—reduce high-glycemic foods.
- Stress reduction.
- Daily fitness levels. This will improve microcirculation.

CONDITION: STAGE II: MODERATE WRINKLES—MODERATE ELASTOSIS— EARLY TO MODERATE PHOTODAMAGE

The first visual signs that you may see with in the client's skin are (Figure 5–7):

- Wrinkles
- Soft sagging jaw line
- Folds of skin above eye
- Double chin
- Sunken cheeks
- Fat pillows under eyes
- Moderate discoloration throughout face
- Dull yellow/gray overall skin tone

Diagnostic Signs

- Moderate-depth wrinkles at rest located around mouth, eyes, forehead, and neck
- **Permanent elastotic creases**, or **static rhytids**: These wrinkles occur in a crisscross pattern and are generally seen on the cheeks and neck. They gradually become permanent.
- Moderate-depth fold at edge of ear when lying down
- Dyschromias and keratosis may be present
- Pronounced hyper- or hypopigmentation
- Dull, rough skin
- Thick coarse skin
- Increased sensitivity
- Elastosis apparent with sagging jaw line, deep nasolabial folds
- Telangiectasias may be present
- Yellow/gray skin tone
- Woods lamp shows deep purple around eyes (elastosis), dark brown spots (epidermal pigment), and light brown spots (dermal pigment)

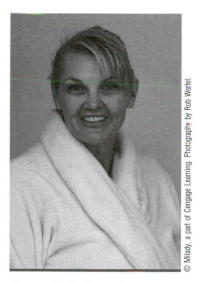

© Milady, a part of Cengage Learning. Photography by Rob Werfel.

Figure 5–7 Stage 2: Moderate wrinkles, elastosis, and early photodamage.

permanent elastotic creases
wrinkles that are present without facial movement.

static rhytids
wrinkles that do not move with facial expression.

Solutions

Esthetic Treatments

Goal: Decrease sensitivity, repair impaired lipid barrier, increase desquamation, increase circulation and lymphatic flow (oxygen transport), reduce TEWL, increase stem cell proliferation, increase antioxidant protection, strengthen facial muscles, decrease melanosome production, and decrease inflammation.

Options:
- Chemical Peeling: Lactic Acid, Glycolic Acid, Enzymes, Modified Jessner's, TCA (>15%)
- Mechanical Exfoliation: Microdermabrasion, Ultrasonic
- Facial Treatments: Focus on antioxidant, peptide, retinol infusion and hydration (hyaluronic acid, ceramides, essential fatty acids), collagen masks, firming masks, mild exfoliation, lymphatic drainage massage, and iontophoresis (galvanic current). Low-level sonophoresis, microcurrent, LED light therapy, microcurrent, new layered anti-aging technology (discussed in Chapter 6).

Medical Treatments

Goal: Stimulate production of collagen, inhibit melanosomes, relax wrinkles, and increase dermal density.

Treatments:
- IPL/photopneumatic
- Ablative lasers
- Fractionated lasers
- Radiofrequency and infrared skin tightening
- Botox
- Dermal filler
- Retinoids
- Medium-depth peel
- Hydroquinone

Professional Products

Cleansers/Toners: Cleanser appropriate to skin type. Toner infused with peptides, antioxidants.

Treatment Products and Moisturizers: Look for some of the following ingredients:

- Ceramides
- Essential fatty acids

- Sphingolipids
- Cholesterol
- Silicones
- Algae
- Hyaluronic acid
- Calcium
- Malus domestica (Phyto Cell Tech)
- Phycosaccharide Al (Phycojuvenine)
- Niacinamide
- Retinaldehyde/Retinol
- Peptides: ALL
- Magnesium ascorbyl phosphate
- Antioxidants: ALL
- Soy
- Pycnogenol
- Beta glucan

Lifestyle Choices

Stage 2 aging is impacted by lifestyle choices. At this stage alcohol, smoking, and lack of sleep should be looked at. The following lifestyle choices need to be addressed;

- Daily intake of water; adequate levels are needed based on body weight and lifestyle.
- Daily UV radiation protection.
- Essential fatty acid deficiency, usually from low-fat diet or chronic dieting or processed food intake.
- Smoking, alcohol intake.
- Diet—reduce high-glycemic foods.
- Stress reduction.
- Daily fitness levels. This will improve microcirculation.
- Adequate sleep.

■ CONDITION: STAGE III: MODERATE TO DEEP WRINKLES—SEVERE ELASTOSIS—SEVERE PHOTODAMAGE

The first visual signs that you may see within the client's skin are (Figure 5–8):

- Deep wrinkles, present without facial movement

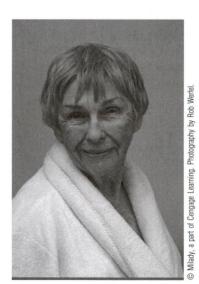

Figure 5–8 Stage 3: Moderate to deep wrinkles, severe elastosis, and photodamage.

- Soft sagging jaw line
- Folds of skin above eye
- Double chin
- Sunken cheeks
- Fat pillows under eyes
- Distinct hyperpigmentation
- Dry rough texture
- Discolorations throughout face

Diagnostic Signs

- **Atrophic crinkling rhytids**: These are fine horizontal and parallel wrinkles that tend to form later in life. They can occur anywhere on the face and body (Figure 5–9).
- **Gravitational fold**, or deep wrinkle: This is a deep groove that is long and straight. It can occur anywhere on the face.
- Keratosis may be present
- Pronounced hyperpigmentation and patches of hypopigmentation are possible
- Telangiectasia present
- Deep fold at outer part of ears when laying down
- Deep nasolabial folds
- Soft sagging jaw line
- Dry, rough skin
- Woods lamp shows excessive sun damage (epidermal—dark brown, dermal—light brown) throughout face
- Yellow/gray skin tone
- Muscle atrophy in cheeks and neck
- Bruises easily

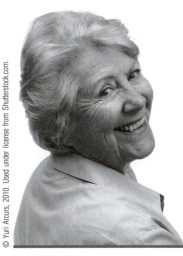

© Yuri Arcurs, 2010. Used under license from Shutterstock.com.

Figure 5–9 Atrophic crinkling wrinkles tend to form later in life.

atrophic crinkling rhytids
fine horizontal and parallel wrinkles that tend to form later in life; they can occur anywhere on the face and body.

gravitational fold
deep wrinkle; this is a deep groove that is long and straight and can occur anywhere on the face.

Solutions

Esthetic Treatments

Goal: Decrease sensitivity, repair impaired lipid barrier, increase desquamation, increase circulation, increase stem cell proliferation, reduce TEWL, strengthen facial muscles, decrease melanosome production, decrease chronic inflammation, and reduce free radical damage. Provide support for aesthetic medical treatments.

Options:
- Chemical Peeling: Lactic Acid, Glycolic Acid, Enzymes, Jessner's, TCA (>15%)

- Mechanical Exfoliation: Microdermabrasion, Ultrasonic
- Facial Treatments: Focus on antioxidant, peptide, retinol infusion and hydration (hyaluronic acid, ceramides, essential fatty acids), collagen masks, firming masks, mild exfoliation, lymphatic drainage massage, and iontophoresis (galvanic current). Low-level sonophoresis, microcurrent, LED light therapy, microcurrent, new layered anti-aging technology (see Chapter 6).

Medical Treatments

Goal: Stimulate production of collagen, inhibit melanosomes, relax wrinkles, increase dermal density, correct muscle and fascia laxity.

Treatments:
- Photopneumatic Therapy (PDT)
- Ablative fractionated lasers
- Ablative laser resurfacing—CO_2
- Rhytidectomy, mid-face lift, eye lift
- Botox
- Dermal filler
- Retinoids
- Medium-depth peel: Azelaic acid
- Hydroquinone

Professional Products

Cleansers/Toners: Focus on gentle, nonsurfactant, neutral pH cleanser.

Treatment Products and Moisturizers: Use the following ingredients:

- Ceramides
- Essential fatty acids
- Sphingolipids
- Cholesterol
- Silicones
- Algae
- Hyaluronic acid
- Calcium
- Niacinamide
- Retinaldehyde/Retinol
- Peptides: ALL

- Magnesium ascorbyl phosphate
- Antioxidants: ALL
- Soy
- Pycnogenol
- Beta glucan

Lifestyle Choices

Stage 3 aging is the result of lifestyle choices and genetics. These recommendations are the same for all aging conditions. The following lifestyle choices need to be addressed:

- Daily intake of water; adequate levels are needed based on body weight and lifestyle.
- Daily UV radiation protection.
- Essential fatty acid deficiency, usually from low-fat diet or chronic dieting.
- Smoking, alcohol intake.
- Diet—reduce high-glycemic foods.
- Stress reduction.
- Daily fitness levels. This will improve microcirculation.
- Adequate sleep.

Adrenocorticotropic hormone (ACTH)
Hormone secreted by the pituitary in response to stress.

POMC (propiomelanocoortin) secreted by the pituitary gland to activate Melanin Stimulating Hormone

melanin stimulating hormone (MSH) responsible for starting the process of pigment creation.

Figure 5–10 Freckled or photo damaged skin.

◾ CONDITION: HYPERPIGMENTATION/ HYPOPIGMENTATION

The first visual signs that you may see within the client's skin are (Figure 5–10):

- Irregular pigmentation throughout face in small brown to dark brown spots
- Gray-colored areas of pigmentation in large spots
- Areas of no pigmentation, usually in small spots

Cause

Melanogenesis is a complicated process which starts with UV radiation or other stimulating factor, such as an increase of **ACTH (adrenocorticotropic) stress hormone** and endocrine disorders.[11]

After the exposure happens then the pituitary gland secretes **POMC (proopiomelanocortin)** in order to activate **MSH (melanin** stimulating hormone). MSH then adheres to a receptor on the melanocyte called **melanocortin**. It is also possible to have the MSH receptor on the keratinocyte start the melanogenesis process, but that is not the primary pathway. The enzyme **tyrosinase** then synthesizes the amino acid tyrosine and L-dopa, dopa phosphates which are the building blocks of melanin, are then activated within the melanocyte to form the **melanosome**, which is the pigment carrier and is an organelle within the cytoplasm of the melanocyte.

Transfer of the melanosome then happens as the melanosome moves along the dendrite tips and up microtubules to come into contact with the keratinocyte and is clear until transfer to the keratinocyte within the spiny layer. See Figure 5–11 for an illustration. The melanosome comes into contact with an average of 36 keratinocytes, which form a melanin unit.[12] The keratinocytes then continue their migration upward to the stratum corneum and help form an integral part of the skin's immune system.

Melanin is responsible for the color in the skin and is the same amount in all skin; it is the size, volume, quality, and degradation of melanin production that accounts for different skin colors. Melanin comes in two types: eumelanin in darker skin and pheomelanin in

melanocortin
a cellular receptor on the melanocyte which Melanin Stimulating Hormone adheres to.

tyrosinase
Enzyme that synthesizes tyrosine and L-DOPA to create the melansome.

melanosome
the organelle of the melanocyte that is the pigment carrier.

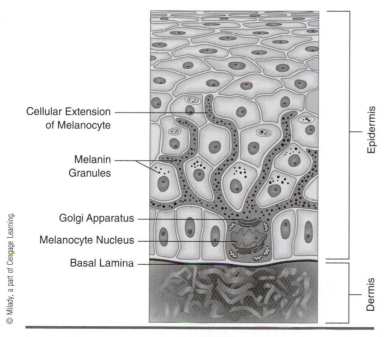

Cellular Extension of Melanocyte

Melanin Granules

Golgi Apparatus

Melanocyte Nucleus

Basal Lamina

Epidermis

Dermis

© Milady, a part of Cengage Learning.

Figure 5–11 An illustration of a melanocyte.

lighter skin. Pigmentation can also be stimulated by photosensitizing medication and topical ingredients.[13,14]

There are several types of pigmentation that an esthetician will see:

- **Melasma:** also known as pregnancy mask, pigmented macules appear over large areas on face. Stimulated by hormonal changes. Also referred to a chloasma.
- **Solar Lentigines:** found in exposed areas of body, usually singular with medium brown to dark coloring. Also referred to as age spots, found to be part of the free radical damage process and are deposited lipofuscins.
- **Ephelides (freckles):** small macules that appear on nose, cheeks, and chin during childhood.
- **Post-Inflammatory Pigmentation:** caused by injury to the dermal or epidermal layer, inflammatory response, and exposure to UV during recovery phase of wound.
- **Polkiderma:** combination of elastin loss, telangiectasia, and hypopigmentation, seen down both sides of neck with clear area under chin.[15]

Diagnostic Signs

- A Woods lamp shows light brown areas (dermal layers) or dark brown areas (epidermal layers) throughout face
- Visible solar lentigines in patches throughout face, especially nose and cheeks
- Loss of pigment (hypopigmentation)

Solutions

Esthetic Treatments

Goal: Prevent MSH stimulation and UV exposure and interrupt phases in the formation of melanin. Epidermal melanin will respond better than dermal melanin.

Options: Pigmentation treatment is highly challenging and requires the commitment of the client to a series of protocols and home treatment.

- **Chemical Peeling:** Lactic acid is a mild tyrosinase inhibitor and will remove affected keratinocytes. Care must be given to not over-stimulate melanosome production. Enzyme exfoliation is effective and gentle.

- **Mechanical Exfoliation:** Microdermabrasion is very effective when used in conjunction with tyrosinase inhibitors.
- **Facial Treatments:** Focus on antioxidant infusion, strengthening the lipid barrier, slowing TEWL, and suppression of tyrosine and melanosomes. In order for pigmentation treatments to be effective the epidermis must be well hydrated, balanced, and protected. Sonophoresis and iontophoresis are effective at infusing the skin with antioxidants; LED light therapy will further strengthen the skin.

Medical Treatments

Goal: Reduce proliferation of melanocytes, inhibit formation of melanosomes, and promote the degradation of melanosomes. Treatments could be:

- IPL (intense pulsed light)
- Nonablative laser (Q-switched)
- Fractionated laser
- Hydroquinone
- Azelaic acid
- Tretinoin
- Medium-depth peels

Professional Products

Daily sunscreen use is mandatory, physical blocks are preferred to reduce inflammation (zinc oxide).

Cleansers/Toners: Cleansers containing enzymes or AHAs. Tonics that deposit tripeptides into skin or reinforce hydration.

Treatment Products and Moisturizers: Use the following ingredients:

- Magnesium ascorbyl phosphate
- Essential fatty acids
- Arbutin
- Glucosamine
- Kojic acid
- Aloesin
- Hyaluronic acid
- Glabridin
- Niacinamide
- Soy

Lifestyle Choices

Pigmentation is affected directly by lifestyle choices such as:

- Daily UV radiation protection.
- Essential fatty acid deficiency, usually from low-fat diet or chronic dieting.
- Smoking, alcohol intake.
- Chronic stress.

▪ SKIN DISORDERS

Skin disorders can show up in any age group. Rosacea is one of the most common disorders to show up in an aging clientele, which can be confused with acne. Acne that is present in an aging skin is usually a resurgence of acne that may have been present in their youth. A disrupted acid mantle can also contribute to an acne flare-up.

Rosacea

Rosacea is one of the most common disorders seen by the esthetician with an aging clientele. It is also very misunderstood, with treatment benefits different for each person. Currently there is no scientific conclusion on what causes rosacea. There are many theories, such as:

- Demodex mites: There are two types of demodex mites, folliculorum and brevis. Folliculorum is implicated in rosacea and lives in the hair follicle.
- Helicobacter pylori infection: It is a common intestinal infection that creates chronic inflammation and is linked to ulcers and stomach cancer.
- Chronic inflammation: It is surmised that an MMP called gelatinase is activated by inflammation and has a direct link to Demodex mites.[16]
- Genetic predisposition

Symptoms:

There are four rosacea subtypes, each with their own set of symptoms:[17]

Subtype 1: Erythematotelangiectatic Rosacea (Figure 5–12)

- Redness in the center of face (cheeks, nose, chin)
- Telangiectasia
- Flushing

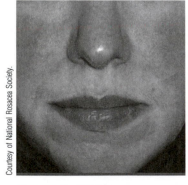

Courtesy of National Rosacea Society.

Figure 5–12 Rosacea subtype 1.

- Aggravated by hot spicy food, hot beverages, alcohol, sunlight, heat
- Sensitive skin

Subtype 2: Papulopustular Rosacea (Figure 5–13)

- Papules
- Pustules
- Persistent erythema on central face (nose, cheeks, chin)
- Aggravated by hot spicy food, hot beverages, alcohol, sunlight, heat
- Often misdiagnosed as acne. If comedones are absent, it is an indicator that it is rosacea.[18]

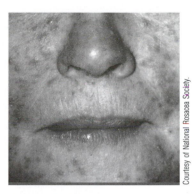

Figure 5–13 Rosacea subtype 2.

Subtype 3: Phymatous Rosacea (Figure 5–14)

- Thick texture on nose
- Irregular surface and nodules on nose

Subtype 4: Ocular Rosacea (Figure 5–15)

- Burning and stinging in eyes
- Telangiectasia on lids
- Sensation of something in eyes
- Red inflamed eyes (often misinterpreted as allergies)

Treatment Modalities:

Treatment options should include a medical approach. This is a progressive disorder that rarely gets better, but esthetic intervention can relieve some of the discomfort if the client is treated while not in a flare. Common medical approaches are:[19]

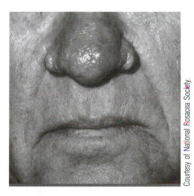

Figure 5–14 Rosacea subtype 3.

Topical Antibiotics:

- Metronidazole
- Clindamycin
- Erythromycin

Topical Immunomodulators:

- Pimecrolimus (Elidel)
- Tacrolimus (Fujimycin)

Topical Anti-inflammatory Ingredients:

- Azelaic acid
- Feverfew
- Green tea
- Licorice extract
- Sulfur

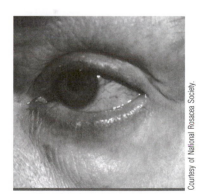

Figure 5–15 Rosacea subtype 4.

Oral Antibiotics:

- Tetracycline
- Ampicillin
- Metronidazole
- Erythromycin
- Clarithromycin

Oral Treatments:

- Isotretinoin (Accutane)
- Aspirin
- Beta-blockers
- Selective serotonin reuptake inhibitors
- Clonidine
- Oral contraceptives

Aesthetic Medical Technology:

- IPL (intense pulsed light)
- Vascular lasers
- CO_2 laser

Esthetic Treatments:

- Enzyme peels
- Glycolic peels
- Hydrating facial treatments with iontophoresis or sonophoresis
- LED light therapy

Professional Products: ingredients should include:

- Retinols
- Topical probiotics
- Olive oil
- Green tea
- Essential fatty acids
- Glycolic acid
- Salicylic acid
- Physical sunscreen (zinc oxide)
- Low level of preservatives

Acne

Acne is a common skin disorder that estheticians deal with. Depending on the grade of acne, a physician will be needed to control the symptoms. This is a disorder that clients will deal with in some manner for most of their lives.

Causes:

1. Excessive sebum production
2. Hyperkeratinization of the cells
3. Inflammation
4. Bacteria
5. Disruption of acid mantle
6. Increased production of androgen hormones

There are four classified types of acne:

Grade 1: open and closed comedomes, may have pustules and papules but no more than 10 lesions on the face.[20]

Grade 2: open and closed comedomes, pustules and papules predominate, 11–25 lesions on each half of face.[21]

Grade 3: inflamed, pustules and papules, open and closed comedomes, may have one cyst or nodule, minimal scarring.[22] Note: *Not to be treated by an esthetician.*

Grade 4: cystic acne, deep nodules, cysts, scarring, open and closed comedomes, severe inflammation.[23] Note: *Not to be treated by an esthetician.*

Medical treatment: many medical modalities are also used by estheticians, except for the pharmaceutical products. Estheticians' additional modalities will be listed in bold.

Normalizing Keratinization

- Tretinoin (Renova, Retin-A, Retin-A micro, Atralin)
- Adapalene (Differin)
- Tazarotene (Tazorac)
- Retinol, retinyl palmitate, retinaldehyde, salicylic acid, **microdermabrasion**
- Oral Isotretinoin (Accutane, Claravis, Sotret, Amnesteen)

Reducing Bacteria

- Topical antibiotics (clindamycin, erythromycin)
- Benzoyl peroxide 2.5%-4%
- Azelaic acid (Azelex)
- **Sulfur-masks and serums**
- Oral antibiotics
- **LED blue light therapy, high frequency**

Remove Hyperkeratinized Cells

- Retinoids
- Salicylic acid

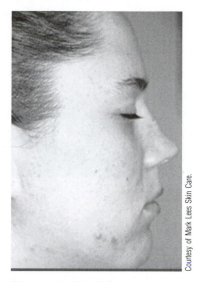

Figure 5–16a The four grades of acne.

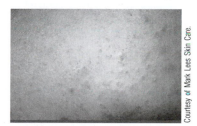

Figure 5–16b

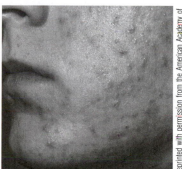

Figure 5–16c

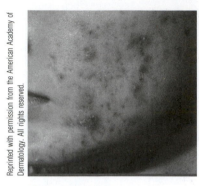

Figure 5–16d

- Alpha hydroxyl acids (glycolic, lactic)
- Azelaic acid
- Microdermabrasion

Reducing Inflammation

- Salicylic acid (topical cleanser, lotion, gel)
- BHA peels
- Oral NSAIDs
- Licorice root extract, colloidal oatmeal

Reducing Sebum Secretions

- Oral contraceptives
- Retinoids
- Essential fatty acids (topically and in diet)
- Beta carotene (topically and in diet)

> The case study client has hyperkeratinization. Note the description of the diagnostic signs on page 89, as these signs can be mistaken for dehydration as well.

Case Study

Let's continue to formulate a plan on our client from Chapter 3, Creating a Healthy Aging Plan. We have done our objective analysis and included subjective information to reach the following conclusions:

Client: 42-year-old female

Skin type: Combination-Fitzpatrick Type 2

Conditions: Photodamage, fine lines (stage 1 aging), dehydration, hyperkeratintization, comedones

Assessment: Client has identified with wrong skin type thus using the wrong home care products, high stress levels are impacting hydration and texture issues in the skin. Perimenopausal symptoms are adding to skin condition. Fitzpatrick type is good for most clinical treatments.

Client Example

Let's put the entire program together.

Skin type: Combination-Fitzpatrick Type 2
Based on the goals of the client, identify the conditions seen within the skin.

Conditions: Stage 1 aging, dehydration, hyperkeratinization
After identifying the conditions seen within the skin, refer to the category indicated and then Esthetic Treatments. The GOAL will be listed under the heading Esthetic Treatments or Medical Treatments. Treatment plans will depend on the esthetician's scope of practice and information that the client is looking for. Thie focus of this client's plan will be based on an esthetic approach. List all of the GOALS for the treatment.

GOALS:

- *increase desquamation*
- *increase free water within epidermis*
- *slow TEWL*
- *increase protection from UVR and free radical damage*

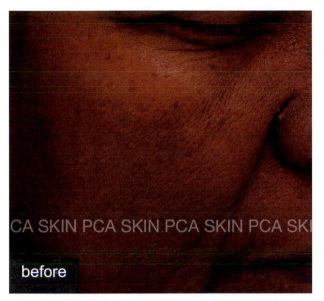
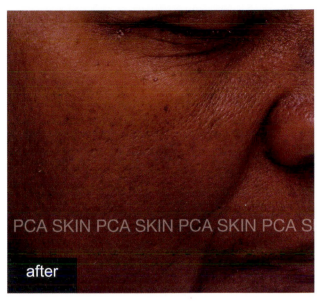

An example of a client's skin before and after using chemical exfoliation for treating hyperpigmentation and rough surface texture

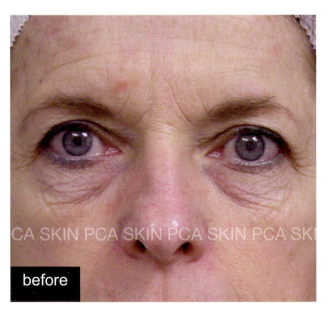
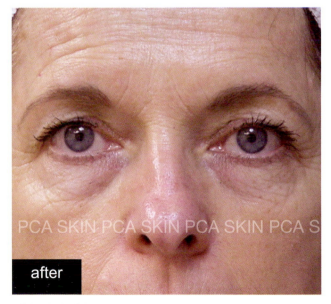

A client with stage 2 aging before and after a series of chemical exfoliation and daily home care.

1. Acid mantle

Function: Maintains a pH of 4.5 to 5.5 on the skin; inhibits growth of harmful bacteria; prevents trans epidermal water loss (TEWL); prevents toxins from being absorbed into skin; promotes the creation of Vitamin D by UV exposure on 7 dehydro cholesterol fatty acid; and acts as a lubricant on surface of skin.

Structure: This layer is actually a complex fluid formed by the excretions from sebaceuous, sodiferious glands, epidermal lipids and NMF (natural moisture factor) and contains 7 dehydrocholesterol fatty acid. This layer has "micro flora" that contributes to the skin's first layer of barrier defense.

2. Stratum corneum

Function: Provides protection; generates the Natural Moisturizing Factor (NMF); regulates moisture balance; and can be up to fifteen (15) cell layers thick on the face. The thickness varies on different parts of the body.

Structure: The Natural Moisturizing Factor (NMF) is created by enzymes breaking down the keratin-fillagrin complex which are protein filiaments that connect keratin and fillagrin together. Lamellar bodies secrete free sterols, sphingolipids, and glycoproteins which allow a balance of both hydrophilic and lipophilic materials to pass through the stratum corneum. Cells in this layer are dead with no nucleus or organelles.

3. Stratum lucidum

Function: Continued formation of the bilayers through the secretion of odland bodies, and the keratinization process continues with keratohylin creating eledin which in turn forms keratin.

Structure: Cells in this layer are dead, having no nucleus and organelles.

4. Stratum granulosm

Function: Responsible for formation of amino acids which create Natural Moisturizing Factor (NMF) and dissolving of the desmosomes.

Structure: Cells have lost their nucleus; structure has started to flatten out.

5. Stratum spinosm

Function: Important to the immune system; cellular changes such as the formation of odland bodies which is a granule that contains ceramide, cholesterol, and free fatty acids start here. Melanocytes synthesize melanin and transfer melansome granules via microtubes to keratinocytes. Aquaporin channels are thought to impact keratinocytes by facilitating transport of water, glycerol and solutes.

Structure: Cells change from columnar structure to polygonal structure which is a shape with no curved sides.

6. Stratum germinativum

Function: Known as basement membrane, or basal layer. Responsible for maintaining the epidermis by continually renewing.

Structure: The dermal papillae (also known as RETE pegs) connect the epidermis to the dermis; melanocytes, langerhan cells, merkel cells and epithelial stem cells are found here. Epithelial cells are shaped like columns.

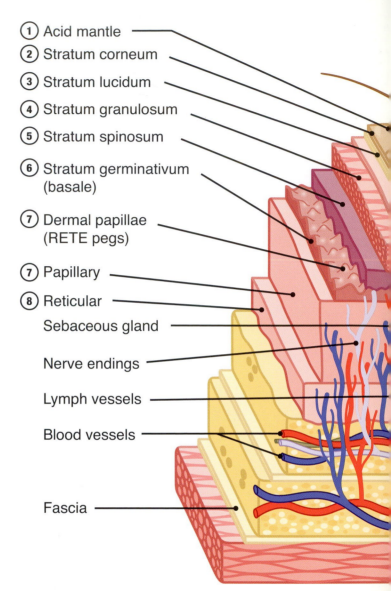

1. Acid mantle
2. Stratum corneum
3. Stratum lucidum
4. Stratum granulosum
5. Stratum spinosum
6. Stratum germinativum (basale)
7. Dermal papillae (RETE pegs)
7. Papillary
8. Reticular
Sebaceous gland
Nerve endings
Lymph vessels
Blood vessels
Fascia

Growth factors such as epiderm to the epidermal growth factor r
- tyrosine kinase activity whi
- keratinocyte growth factor hyaluronan synthesis, cell wound healing.

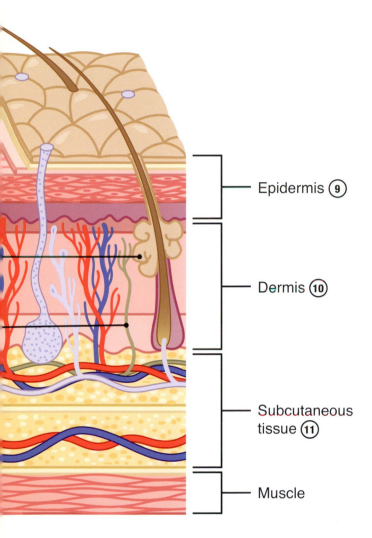

Epidermis ⑨

Dermis ⑩

Subcutaneous tissue ⑪

Muscle

7. Papillary layer

Function: At the top of the papillary layer is the dermal/ epidermal junction, also known as dermal papilla or RETE ridges. This area connects the dermis and epidermis together and helps provide the epidermal cells with oxygen and nutrients from blood as well as hydration from the lymph capillaries.

Structure: Most active layer of the dermis and is made up of loose collagen and elastin fibers known as areolar surrounded by glycosaminoglycans, (GAG's) well as mast cells, phagocytes, white blood cells, fibroblasts and fibrocytes. Blood, lymph vessels, sebaceous, sudoriferous glands, nerves and shafts of hair follicles are also are found throughout the dermis.

8. Reticular layer

Function: This layer is important for cell to cell signaling, wound repair, cell adhesion, positioning, proliferation, and identity. Fibroblasts are responsible for creating the ground substance as well as maintaining it.

Structure: Found under the papillary layer of the dermis; contains ground substance which surrounds all the cells of the dermis and gives shape and structure to the dermis. Dense type III collagen is found here.

9. Epidermis

Function: The outermost layer of the skin; acts as a thin protective covering with many nerve endings.

Structure: The epidermis is composed of five strata (layers): stratum corneum, stratum lucidum, stratum granulosm, stratum spinosm, and stratum germinativum (basal layer).

10. Dermis

Function: The live layer of connective tissues below the epidermis and acts as a support structure and nourishes the lower epidermis.

Structure: The dermis is comprised of two layers: the papillary layer and the reticular layer. It contains connective tissues made of collagen protein and elastin fibers, as well as blood and lymph vessels.

11. Subcutaneous tissue

Function: The subcutaneous tissue creates a protective cushion that gives contour and smoothness to the body, while also providing a source of energy to the body.

Structure: The subcutaneous tissue is located beneath the dermis.

al growth factor (EGF) bind ceptor (EGFR) and activates: results in cell proliferation (KGF) which enhances proliferation, and enhances

Also present in the basal layer are polypeptide growth factors; TGF-a and TGF-b, protoeoglycans and collagen types IV and VII.
- TGF-a stimulates the tyrosine kinase activity.
- TGF-b promotes cell differentiation and is shown to have role in scarring.

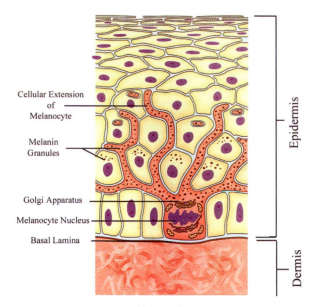

Cellular Extension
of
Melanocyte

Melanin
Granules

Golgi Apparatus

Melanocyte Nucleus

Basal Lamina

Epidermis

Dermis

Melanocytes

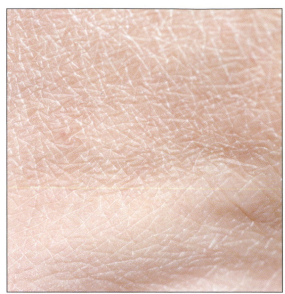

Example of dehydrated skin. Lifestyle factors can effect
this skin, as well as incorrect home care.

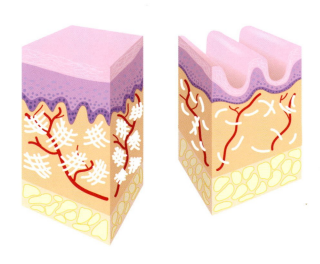

Old and young skin

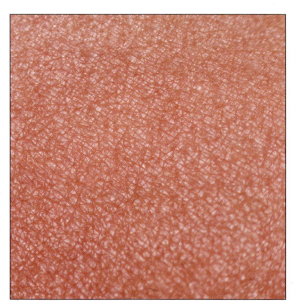

Rough skin can be treated with enzyme and acid peels.

- *increase fibroblast stimulation*
- *decrease glycation*
- *reduce lipid peroxidation*
- *increase antioxidant protection*
- *increase microcirculation and lymphatic flow (oxygenation of the skin)*
- *increase stem cell proliferation*
- *slow MMP activation*

After identifying all GOALS for treatment, list all treatment options available, from esthetic treatments to changes in lifestyle habits.

Professional Treatments:

- *Facial Treatments: (2 options)*
- *Focus on hydration of skin (hyaluronic acid, ceramides, and essential fatty acids), mild exfoliation, stimulating massage (unless sensitivity is present), lymphatic drainage massage, and iontophoresis (galvanic current).*
- *Focus on antioxidant infusion and hydration (hyaluronic acid, ceramides, algae, and essential fatty acids), mild exfoliation, lymphatic drainage massage, firming compression masks, and iontophoresis (galvanic current). Low-level sonophoresis, microcurrent, LED light therapy.*
- *Chemical Peeling: Lactic Acid, Glycolic Acid, Enzymes, Modified Jessner's*
- *Mechanical Exfoliation: Microdermabrasion, Ultrasonic*

Professional Products: Sunscreen daily is mandatory to prevent further damage. (SPF 30+).
Cleansers/Toners: *Appropriate for skin type, possibly with a mild AHA or enzyme. Tonic with peptides or focusing on increasing water content in stratum corneum.*
Treatment Products and Moisturizers: *Look some of the following ingredients:*

- *Ceramides*
- *Essential fatty acids*
- *Sphingolipids*
- *Silicones*
- *Algae*
- *Hyaluronic acid*
- *Calcium*
- *Niacinamide*
- *Retinaldehyde/Retinol*
- *Peptides: wrinkle smoothing, pigment inhibitors, antioxidant*
- *Magnesium ascorbyl phosphate*
- *Antioxidants: ALL*
- *Soy*
- *Pycnogenol*
- *Malus domestica (Phyto Cell Tech)*
- *Phycosaccharide AI (Phycojuvenine)*
- *Beta glucan*
- *Arbutin*
- *Paper mulberry*

Lifestyle Choices

- *Daily intake of water; adequate levels are needed based on body weight and lifestyle.*
- *Daily UV radiation protection.*
- *Essential fatty acid deficiency, usually from low-fat diet or chronic dieting.*
- *Smoking, alcohol intake.*
- *Diet—reduce high-glycemic foods.*
- *Stress reduction.*
- *Daily fitness levels. This will improve microcirculation.*

After listing options available for treatment, refer to the client's healthy aging consultation to determine what modalities may be appropriate.

Assessment: Client has identified with wrong skin type, thus using the wrong home care products. High stress levels are impacting hydration and texture issues in the skin. Perimenopausal symptoms are adding to skin condition. Fitzpatrick type is good for most clinical treatments.

Lifestyle Assessment: Daily fitness is good; diet and water intake may be lacking due to travel and stress. Consistency with self-care and home use of professional products lacking. A program designed around ease of use will be important.

Based on this client's assessment an esthetic plan that has a focus on the following will be appropriate:

Professional Treatments: Results-oriented treatments that also induce the relaxation response will be important. Shorter-duration treatments with high impact such as microdermabrasion will be indicated when client's travel schedule increases. See Chapter 6 for more details.

- *Facial Treatments: focus on antioxidant infusion and hydration (hyaluronic acid, ceramides, algae, and essential fatty acids), mild exfoliation, lymphatic drainage massage, firming compression masks, and iontophoresis (galvanic current). Low-level sonophoresis, microcurrent, LED light therapy.*
- *Chemical Peeling: Lactic Acid, Glycolic Acid, Enzymes*
- *Mechanical Exfoliation: Microdermabrasion, Ultrasonic*

Professional Products: Products with an emphasis on hydration, protection, and ease of use is the first place to start in home care. Dual-purpose products are effective, such as a moisturizer with SPF and gentle cleanser with proteolytic enzymes. See Chapter 7 for more details.

Treatment products should be focused on anti-aging ingredients, stable sun protection, and antioxidants such as:

- *Retinol*
- *Antioxidants—ergothioneine, vitamin C*
- *Alpha lipoic acid*
- *Ceramides*
- *Hyaluronic acid*
- *Peptides*

Lifestyle Choices: This portion of the healthy aging plan is dependant on the commitment of the client. General guidance can be given as well as referrals to other professionals. See Chapters 9–11 for additional information. Some advice to be given to this client could be:

Increase water intake

Daily supplementation: fish oil 2000 mg, D3 1000mg, antioxidant blend

Diet: decrease simple carbohydrates, increase protein (if dieting, one plan is to intake 1 gram of protein based on the desired weight; i.e., 150 pounds goal=150 grams of protein)

Fitness: yoga (stress reduction, strength building), weight training (increases strength, HGH, and metabolism and decreases stress).

Initially putting together a client's healthy aging plan can be complicated but very satisfying as your client sees the improvement in their skin and feels the increased wellness.

⟩ ⟩ ⟩ Top Ten Tips to Take to the Clinic

1. Understand the layers of the skin and their functions at the cellular level.
2. Start the skin assessment with subjective symptoms, then move to objective conditions.
3. List all objective conditions first, then match to listed skin conditions per category.
4. Design a treatment plan based on the most apparent conditions first, with a focus on the client's initial concern.
5. Utilize advanced diagnostic tools such as a Woods lamp.
6. Incorporate lifestyle changes and recommendations in program.
7. Understand and inform the client about possible medical aesthetic treatment options.
8. Explain the physiology of the skin and how the condition has happened; this will give the client realistic expectations.
9. Always recommend and have available a good selection of UV protection for daily use.
10. Learn the signs and symptoms of skin disorders such as rosacea and acne, and always refer clients to a dermatologist.

Chapter Review Questions

1. What is the function of the acid mantle?
2. What is the function of the stratum granulosum?
3. What is the function of the stratum basale?
4. What are the diagnostic signs of stage 1 aging skin?
5. What are the subtypes of rosacea?

References

1. Barrett-Hill, F. (2004). *Advanced Skin Analysis*, 2nd Edition. Whangaparaoa, New Zealand: Virtual Beauty Corporation Ltd.
2. Baumann, L. MD., Saghari, S. MD., Weisburg, E. MS. (2009). *Cosmetic Dermatology: Principles and Practice*, 2nd Edition. New York: McGraw Hill Medical.
3. Pugliese, P. MD. (2001). *Physiology of the Skin II*. Carol Stream, IL: Allured Publishing.

4. Pugliese, P. MD. (2001). *Physiology of the Skin II*. Carol Stream, IL: Allured Publishing.

5. Pugliese, P. MD. (2001). *Physiology of the Skin II*. Carol Stream, IL: Allured Publishing.

6. Barrett-Hill, F. (2004). *Advanced Skin Analysis*, 2nd Edition. Whangaparaoa, New Zealand: Virtual Beauty Corporation Ltd.

7. Thornfeldt, C. MD., Bourne, K. LE. (2010). *The New Ideal in Skin Health: Separating Fact from Fiction*. Carol Stream, IL: Allured Publishing.

8. Baumann, L. MD., Saghari, S. MD., Weisburg, E. MS. (2009). *Cosmetic Dermatology: Principles and Practice*, 2nd Edition. New York: McGraw Hill Medical.

9. Thornfeldt, C. MD., Bourne, K. LE. (2010). *The New Ideal in Skin Health: Separating Fact from Fiction*. Carol Stream, IL: Allured Publishing.

10. Baumann, L. MD., Saghari, S. MD., Weisburg, E. MS. (2009). *Cosmetic Dermatology: Principles and Practice*, 2nd Edition. New York: McGraw Hill Medical.

11. Baumann, L. MD., Saghari, S. MD., Weisburg, E. MS. (2009). *Cosmetic Dermatology: Principles and Practice*, 2nd Edition. New York: McGraw Hill Medical.

12. Baumann, L. MD., Saghari, S. MD., Weisburg, E. MS. (2009). *Cosmetic Dermatology: Principles and Practice*, 2nd Edition. New York: McGraw Hill Medical.

13. Baumann, L. MD., Saghari, S. MD., Weisburg, E. MS. (2009). *Cosmetic Dermatology: Principles and Practice*, 2nd Edition. New York: McGraw Hill Medical.

14. Barrett-Hill, F. (2004). *Advanced Skin Analysis*, 2nd Edition. Whangaparaoa, New Zealand: Virtual Beauty Corporation Ltd.

15. Baumann, L. MD., Saghari, S. MD., Weisburg, E. MS. (2009). *Cosmetic Dermatology: Principles and Practice*, 2nd Edition. New York: McGraw Hill Medical.

16. Baumann, L. MD., Saghari, S. MD., Weisburg, E. MS. (2009). *Cosmetic Dermatology: Principles and Practice*, 2nd Edition. New York: McGraw Hill Medical.

17. Baumann, L. MD., Saghari, S. MD., Weisburg, E. MS. (2009). *Cosmetic Dermatology: Principles and Practice*, 2nd Edition. New York: McGraw Hill Medical.

18. Baumann, L. MD., Saghari, S. MD., Weisburg, E. MS. (2009). *Cosmetic Dermatology: Principles and Practice*, 2nd Edition. New York: McGraw Hill Medical.

19. Baumann, L. MD., Saghari, S. MD., Weisburg, E. MS. (2009). *Cosmetic Dermatology: Principles and Practice*, 2nd Edition. New York: McGraw Hill Medical.
20. Thornfeldt, C. MD., Bourne, K. LE. (2010). *The New Ideal in Skin Health: Separating Fact from Fiction*. Carol Stream, IL: Allured Publishing.
21. Thornfeldt, C. MD., Bourne, K. LE. (2010). *The New Ideal in Skin Health: Separating Fact from Fiction*. Carol Stream, IL: Allured Publishing.
22. Thornfeldt, C. MD., Bourne, K. LE. (2010). *The New Ideal in Skin Health: Separating Fact from Fiction*. Carol Stream, IL: Allured Publishing.
23. Thornfeldt, C. MD., Bourne, K. LE. (2010). *The New Ideal in Skin Health: Separating Fact from Fiction*. Carol Stream, IL: Allured Publishing.

Bibliography

Barrett-Hill, F. (2010). *Cosmetic Chemistry*. Whangaparaoa, New Zealand: Virtual Beauty Corporation Ltd.

Culp, J., et al. (2010). *Milady's Standard Esthetics: Advanced*, 1st Edition. Clifton Park, NY: Milady Cengage Learning.

Lees, Mark PHD. (2001). *Skin Care: Beyond the Basics*. New York: Thompson Delmar Learning.

Websites

www.rosacea.net
www.emedicine.com
www.yglabs.com

Esthetic Treatment Options

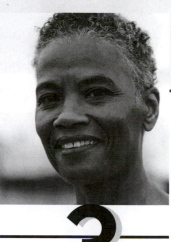

Section **3**

Esthetic Treatments

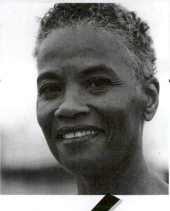

Chapter 6

Key Terms

anion

anode

cathode

cation

cavitation

dyschromia

electrolytes

extraction

homeostasis

hyperpigmentation

ionized solution

iontophoresis

keratin (keratinized)

lacunae

manual lymphatic
   drainage

negative pole

piezoelectric effect

positive pole

rhytids

saponification

sonophoresis

telangiectasia

vasoconstrictive

vasodilative

Learning Objectives

After completing this chapter, you will be able to:

1. Explain the purpose of each phase of the professional esthetic treatment.

2. Design an effective treatment for the healthy aging client.

3. Apply healthy aging makeup techniques.

4. Describe esthetic technology used in healthy aging treatments.

INTRODUCTION

Esthetic treatments are the core of the healthy aging plan. Esthetic treatments can be considered an art and science that require a great deal of flexibility when working with clients. This chapter gives general guidelines of the esthetic modalities available to treat various aging conditions. When looking at how to treat aging skin, you should link the functions of the different epidermal layers to the type of treatment.

Chapter 5 covered the most common conditions, with details on how the physiology of the skin is impacted. Now we will link those conditions to various treatments; for example, a hyperkeratinized skin requires a multi-therapeutic approach with an esthetic treatment that will focus on exfoliation. It is not enough just to exfoliate; the esthetician must choose the correct process based on the skin's physiology. In this case a process that affects the desmosomes as well as increasing hydration is the best approach.

FACIAL TREATMENTS

Every manufacturer has specific protocols for facial treatments, and it is important for an esthetician to be knowledgeable when using products. It is not enough just to apply products as directed; it is important to understand how each phase of a facial treatment is designed to affect the skin.

There are many ways of performing esthetic treatments. This industry is diverse, with many interesting and effective ways of treating skin. An esthetician will have to try hard to become bored.

One of the most common approaches in American esthetics is the theory of stimulation and sedation within a facial treatment. This approach is believed to be introduced by the father of American esthetics, the late Robert Diemer, who also introduced the professional skin analysis system that many estheticians have been trained on.

The purpose of this approach is to increase microcirculation in the stimulation phase in order to activate the skin's self-cleansing and to cause vasoconstriction in the sedation phase in order to activate the skin's self-healing, regenerating process. Many estheticians have built on this theory since the 1970s.

The beginning of the facial is the stimulation phase; the massage starts the sedation phase (Figure 6–1). The results can be dramatic when techniques are applied properly.

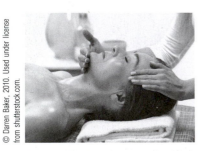

Figure 6–1 A client receiving a facial treatment.

Cleansing–Stimulation Phase

The beginning of the esthetic treatment is always the first cleanse (Figure 6–2). This step utilizes a product that will remove the client's makeup or first layer of debris on the stratum corneum. The first cleanse is done before the skin analysis, and a makeup remover should be used.

Purpose:

Removal of debris from stratum corneum for clear analysis of skin and to prep the skin for second cleansing.

Used for:

All skin types and conditions.

Desired Results:

Clean balanced skin.

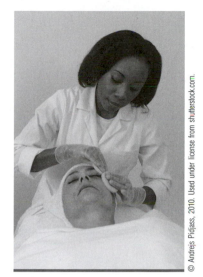

Figure 6–2 The cleansing phase removes makeup and the first layer of debris.

Cleansing–The Second Cleanse

The next step is the second cleanse, which will utilize a cleansing product determined by the skin analysis.

Purpose:

Deep cleanse skin with product based on skin type and condition.

Used for:

All skin types.

Desired Results:

Remove deeply imbedded debris, increase microcirculation, maintain neutral pH.

Toning–Stimulation and Sedation Phases

The toning phase is used throughout the facial treatment to infuse active ingredients, adjust the pH of the stratum corneum, exfoliate, soothe irritation, and hydrate or help kill bacteria depending on the type of product or equipment used. Common examples of equipment used are the Lucas spray (Figure 6–3), vacuum spray machine, and CO_2 spray.

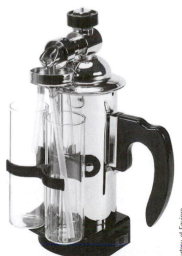

Figure 6–3 A Lucas spray hydrates, soothes, and tones the skin.

Table 6–1 Common toners and tonics and their uses.

Types of Toners and Tonics	Skin Type and Conditions to Treat
Hydrating Toner	Dehydration, hyperkeratinization, sensitivity
pH Balancing Toner	All skin types, sensitivity, dehydration
Tonic	Deposit active ingredients in aging skin, sensitivity, uneven skin tone
Astringent	Uses acidic pH to kill bacteria, balance oily skin types, treat acne

Purpose:

To hydrate, soothe, exfoliate, adjust pH, infuse active ingredients, and suppress bacteria. It is common to use a toner in the stimulation phase and a tonic to deposit active ingredients into the skin in the sedation phase.

Used for:

All skin types (refer to Table 6–1 for a chart of common toners and tonics and their uses).

Exfoliation—Stimulation Phase

Exfoliation is an important aspect of esthetic treatments. There are two options available:

1. Physical: manual scrubs, microdermabrasion, ultrasonic tool
2. Chemical: acids (BHA, AHA), enzymes (for example, papain, bromelain)

Purpose:

Remove the stratum corneum in a controlled manner to activate the skin's wound healing response.

Used for:

All skin types. Modality should be chosen based on skin condition. For example, sensitive skin should not be treated with a manual scrub. Refer to Table 6–2 for a chart detailing the types of exfoliation.

Desired Results:

Removal of stratum corneum to facilitate penetration of active ingredients, soften texture, stimulate healing response within the dermis which

Table 6–2 Chart of types of exfoliation and when to use them.

Types of Exfoliation	Skin Types and Conditions to Treat
AHA–Lactic acid–mild tyrosinase inhibitor, safe for all Fitzpatrick types, hydrophilic (attracted to water)	Hyperpigmentation, stage 1–2 aging, combination, dry skin, dehydration
AHA–Glycolic acid–small molecular size, hydrophilic (attracted to water), safe for most Fitzpatrick types at a percentage less than 30	Stage 1–3 aging, hyperkeratinized skin, hyperpigmentation
BHA–Salicylic acid–lipophilic (attracted to oil)	Acne, oily skin, comedones, milia, hyperpigmentation
Scrubs–increase microcirculation, remove stratum corneum, depth can be controlled somewhat	Hyperkeratinization, oily, congested, dull, dehydrated
Proteolytic Enzymes–dissolve dead skin cells, reduce inflammation, facilitate easier extraction, usually use papain and bromolain	All skin types and conditions

© Milady, a part of Cengage Learning.

activates stem cells, break desmosomes to increase movement of keratinocytes, lighten pigmentation, and increase hydration.

Extraction–Stimulation Phase

Extraction is not used with every treatment but is vital when treating acne or other impacted skin (Figure 6–4). Tools used are extractors, lancets, and desincrustation mediums, such as baking soda and water or other manufacturer blends. Technology used is galvanic current on the negative pole to create saponification.

Purpose:

Expression of comedones, microcomedones, pustules, and milia.

Used for:

All skin types with comedones, milia.

Desired Results:

Less congested skin, removal of milia and comedones.

extraction
technique used to remove comedones, milia, and pustules from skin. Tools and manual pressure may be used.

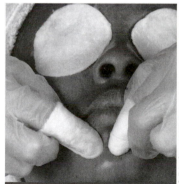

© Tyler Olson, 2010. Used under license from shutterstock.com.

Figure 6–4 Extractions remove comedones, pustules, and milia.

There is debate in the massage and esthetic communities about where an esthetician can massage. In the traditional esthetics training an esthetician is trained as a massage therapist as well. Only in the United States are the two fields separated. Many massage therapists are estheticians as well. The reality is that the massage techniques used during a facial treatment are different than those used during a massage therapy service. The focus for the esthetic model is to promote the strengthening, hydration, and lymph capillary movement within the skin, not just focus on the muscle. Both are valuable approaches and should be seen as complementary, not competitive.

manual lymphatic drainage (MLD) massage technique used to move lymph fluid to lymph nodes.

Massage–Sedation Phase

Massage is one of the most beneficial steps in the esthetic treatment process and has multiple benefits based on type of massage used, amount of time performed, as well as the massage medium used. This is the one modality that all estheticians should master.

Purpose:

Increase microcirculation to bring oxygen and nutrients to cells, induce the relaxation response, improve lymph circulation for removal of toxins as well as increasing epidermal hydration (free water content), stimulate cellular function, aid in desquamation, stimulate sebaceous glands, and facilitate penetration of active ingredients.

Used for:

All skin types, essential for aging skin conditions; avoid facial massage after aggressive exfoliation treatments. Incorporate the use of toning movements if the skin is losing elasticity, important in stage 3–4 aging. Do not overstimulate skin with rosacea or acne. There are specialized massage techniques that the esthetician can learn that directly treat aging skin. **Manual lymphatic drainage** of the face is one of the most useful. This does require extensive additional training. Refer to Table 6–3 for identifying types of massage for particular skin types and conditions.

Desired Results:

Reduction of subclinical inflammation through increased lymph circulation, reduction in stress hormones and penetration of actives, smoother, softer skin texture, and healthy glow.

Infusion of Active Ingredients–Sedation Phase

Infusion of active ingredients is done through the application of serums and ampoules as well as utilizing technology such as galvanic current, ultrasound, and electroporation. Massage facilitates this process and care should be taken to determine when to apply the serum. A lipid-based serum does well after the massage phase and before the mask. A water-based serum is often used before the massage to facilitate hydration in the epidermis. See Chapter 7 for more information on active ingredients and their uses.

Table 6–3 Types of massage for skin conditions.

Types of Massage Used in Facial Treatments	Skin Types and Conditions to Treat
Effleurage–sedating and relaxing effect, can be superficial or deep movements, aids in desquamation, reduces edema, and increases microcirculation and lymph flow.	All skin types Contraindicated for: acne grades 2–4, rosacea
Petrissage–lifting, rolling, knuckling, varied pressure, helps tone, and stimulates microcirculation and lymph flow, improves elasticity.	All aging skin conditions, all skin types Contraindicated for: acne grades 2–4, rosacea. Jacquet movements for non-inflamed acne grade 1.
Tapotement–a light tapping feathering motion, increases microcirculation and lymph flow, improves muscle tone.	Aging skin conditions stage 2–3
Lymphatic Drainage–feather-light, wave-like movements along the lymphatic channels, moves fluid, reduces puffiness, aids in healing. Important post-surgery.	All skin types
Facelift Massage–a combination of techniques that can include acupressure points, deep contouring lifting movements, tapotement, lymph drainage and hot stones, spoons or other items. Done in a series of 6–12 treatments, once a week.	All types except acne. Specific to aging skin stages 1–3.

© Milady, a part of Cengage Learning.

Purpose:

To introduce specific ingredients into the epidermis that will influence specific cellular reactions within the skin.

Used for:

Specific skin conditions such as loss of firmness, dehydration, hyperpigmentation, blemishes, lines, wrinkles, and sensitivity.

Desired Results:

Improvement of conditions in the skin through enhanced cellular processes, reduction of inflammation, increased barrier repair.

Masking–Sedation Phase

The masking phase of the esthetic treatment utilizes several different types of products. Masks can be clay based, emollient based, or occlusive such as paraffin. The benefits of a mask are determined by the type and duration left on skin. Depending on the temperature of the mask used on the skin, the microcirculation will be increased or decreased. This effect helps nutrients pass into the epidermis as well as increase lymphatic capillary diffusion and stimulates the sudorferous glands to secrete. Occlusion and heat are also used to help make active ingredients penetrate the stratum corneum. Compression masks act on the skin by moving interstitial fluid within the skin for a sculpting effect as well as activating fibroblasts within the dermis.

Purpose:

Masks are used to treat the stratum corneum (exfoliate, hydrate), help active ingredients penetrate, and increase or decrease microcirculation within the skin.

Used for:

All skin types and conditions. Refer to Table 6–4 for the mask types and skin conditions that certain masks treat.

Desired Results:

Even tone, improved texture, increased hydration, increased penetration of active ingredients applied underneath.

Moisture Replacement and Protection–Sedation Phase

Moisture replacement and protection is the finishing phase of every esthetic treatment. Improving and maintaining the skin's protective barrier is a vital part of skin health. An impaired barrier leads to TEWL (transepidermal water loss), inflammation, and impaired acid mantle, which lead to reduced immune response.

Protection refers to applying an SPF protection cream to the skin. The minimum SPF used should be SPF 15 and needs to be a broad spectrum protection. Broad spectrum protection refers to a sunscreen that provides both UVA and UVB protection.

Purpose:

To help repair an impaired barrier, protect against UV radiation, and reduce inflammation.

> Cold temperature will decrease microcirculation and warm temperatures will increase microcirculation.

Table 6-4 Different mask types and the skin conditions treated.

Types of Masks	Skin Types and Conditions to Treat
CLAY/MINERAL MUD	
Kaolin–aluminum silicate mineral, color depends on iron oxides and aluminum content. Gentle, *does not* draw oils from skin but does have some absorbent properties[1]	Dry, aging, oily, combination skin
Bentonite–volcanic ash sediment, 70 trace elements and montmorillonite, absorbent	Oily, combination skin
Fuller's Earth–sedimentary clay with alumina, silica, iron oxides, lime, and magnesium. Absorbent, increases microcirculation, draws excess sebaceous secretions from skin	Oily, acne skin
Green Clay–decomposed plant matter, trace minerals, microalgae, kelp. Stimulates microcirculation, absorbs impurities, and exfoliates	All skin types
Rhassoul Clay (Moroccan clay)–high percentage of silica, magnesium, calcium, potassium. Minerals acclimate easily due to keratinocyte receptors for elements in clay	All skin types
Dead Sea Mud–high concentration of minerals. Soothing, healing, and hydrating	Sensitive, dehydrated, aging, dry skin
Moor Mud (Austria/peloid)–over 1,000 different herbs, organic substances, minerals, trace elements, and vitamins. Soothing, healing, and hydrating	All skin types, dehydrated, aging
GEL–water-based mask infused with active ingredients such as minerals and trace elements. Hydrating, calming	All skin types, dehydrated, aging, acne
CRÈME–emollient-based mask, can be mixed with clays. Provides occlusion and hydration	Dry, combination, aging, dehydrated skin
PLASTER–occlusive mask mixed with water to provide compression and occlusion on the surface of skin	All skin types except acne, sensitive skin
ALGINATE–soft occlusive mask with algae base, rubber texture, provides mild compression and hydration	All skin types
COMPRESSION–mask designed to compress tissue to move fluid causing a temporary tightening of skin. Ingredients may include egg white and algae, usually in powder form	All skin types
PARAFFIN–warm wax applied for occlusive effect, increases hydration in epidermis	All skin types except acne and sensitive

Used for:

All skin types.

Desired Results:

Smoother skin texture, reduction in fine lines, even color.

Creating a Healthy Aging Treatment

When first considering a facial protocol, start by determining the genetic skin type, the client's healing response time, and contraindications to treatment. Refer to Chapter 5 for an example on how to start the consultation process. After the initial intake forms are filled out, the analysis process can continue. It is a good idea to first address the client's most important concern. Many concerns that clients have are really manifestations of other diagnostic issues that can be addressed throughout the treatment program.

Most professional esthetic product manufacturers have a basic hydrating facial protocol that the esthetician can rely on when first consulting with a client. To customize an esthetic treatment based on specific conditions requires a little more thought but can be done easily with an understanding of the purpose of each phase of treatment as well as knowledge of the product line used. See Table 6–5 on page 129. for treatment goals and esthetic treatment options for an easy reference.

Here is an example of designing a treatment for the skin condition dehydration, also known as fast TEWL, with a genetic skin type of oily and Fitzpatrick type 2. Start with identifying the goal for this skin.

Example

Goal:

Increase free water within the skin, slow TEWL through barrier repair, replace lost lipids, and remove stratum corneum for better ingredient infusion.

Based on these goals and the purpose of each phase, the treatment would look like this:

Stimulation Phase

Cleansing:

First cleansing done with a makeup remover or gel cleanser, second cleanse done with a gel cleanser created for oily skin.

> After the goal of the treatment is determined, look at the purpose of each phase for the direction in which to proceed. For example, slowing TEWL would be associated with the moisture and infusion phases. Referring to Chapter 5 you will see that TEWL is greatly impacted by lifestyle, environment, and the acid mantle of the skin. This helps the esthetician plan the treatment with a focus on acid mantle repair to slow TEWL.

Table 6–5 Chart of treatment goals and esthetic options.

Goal	Common Visual Signs	Phase of Treatment	Treatment Goals and Esthetic Options
Increase desquamation/ dead cell turnover	Hyperkeratinization-dead skin cell buildup, comedones, milia	Exfoliation, cleansing, massage	Enzymes, AHA acids, BHA acids, blended peels, scrubs, exfoliating masks, cleanser with acids, microdermabrasion, ultrasonic, brush machine or sonic brush, stimulating massage movements
Increase free water in epidermis/ hydration, slow TEWL	Dehydration, impaired acid mantle, flakey, erythema	Toner, active ingredient infusion, massage, moisturize and protect, mask	Hydrating serums, toners, humectant moisturizer, hydrating mask, penetration w/galvanic current, sonophoresis, massage general movements, facelift massage
Increase micro-circulation, lymphatic flow, oxygenation absorbtion	Dull sallow color, telangiectasia, hyperkeratinization, comedones, milia	Massage, cleansing, infusion of active ingredients	Facelift massage, MLD massage, stimulating massage movements, cleansing under steam, oxygenating serums
Increase protection from UV and free radicals	Hyper/hypopigmentation, loss of elasticity, hyperkeratinization, dehydration	Moisturize and protect, infusion of active ingredients	Antioxidant serums, moisturizer, sun protection
Increase fibroblast stimulation	Fine lines and wrinkles, loss of elasticity	Exfoliation, infusion of active ingredients	Enzyme exfoliation, acid peels, microderma-brasion, ultrasonic, galvanic current (iontophoresis)
Decrease glycation	Fine lines, rough texture	Infusion of active ingredients	Serums with alpha lipoic acid, vitamins, antioxidants
Reduce inflammation	Subclinical—no visible signs except accelerated aging, possible sensitivity	Cleansing, toning, infusion of active ingredients	Cleansers/toners used for sensitive skin, dry skin, active ingredient infusion, galvanic current, microcurrent, MLD massage
Slow MMP activation	Loss of elasticity	Protection, infusion of active ingredients, massage	Active ingredient infusion w/sonophoresis, galvanic current, massage
Reduce sensitivity	Impaired acid mantle, dehydration, flakey, erythema	Cleansing, toning, infusion of active ingredients, mask	Cleansers/toners used for sensitive skin, colloidal oatmeal mask, hydrating gel mask
Strengthen facial muscles	Sagging	Massage	Specialized massage techniques—facelift massage

© Milady, a part of Cengage Learning.

(continued)

Table 6–5 Chart of treatment goals and esthetic options. (*Continued*)

Goal	Common Visual Signs	Phase of Treatment	Treatment Goals and Esthetic Options
Inhibit tyrosinase production, slow melanosome transfer	Hyperpigmentation, uneven skin tone	Infusion of active ingredients, toning	Serums containing melanin suppressants, galvanic current, sonophoresis, massage
Repair impaired lipid barrier—essential fatty acid deficiency	Dehydration, erythema, flakey, sensitive, comedones, milia	Massage, infusion of active ingredients, moisturize and protect	Massage w/lipid-rich medium, galvanic current, sonophoresis, microcurrent
Stimulate stem cell proliferation	Aging skin	Exfoliation, infusion of active ingredients	AHA/BHA, Jessner's, TCA peels, microdermabrasion, infusion of active ingredients w/galvanic, microcurrent, sonophoresis

Toning:

Toning phase is done with an astringent to start to remove the stratum corneum and make pH slightly acidic.

Exfoliation:

This client is a Fitzpatrick type 2; keep the exfoliation mild until the skin is properly prepped. Chemical peel done with a designer peel blend of multiple AHAs and salicylic acid, no higher than 30 percent or pH of less than 3.5. Use manufacturer directions to assure full neutralization of solution. See Chapter 7 for additional information on professional products.

Sedation Phase

You will notice that the active ingredient infusion is after the exfoliation step, and this is due to the focus of the treatment—dehydration. Massage is usually done with a lipid-rich medium, active ingredients are usually a smaller molecular structure and in a water base. It will be easier to get the active ingredients into the skin when they are applied first.

Toning:

Toning phase is done with gentle hydrating toner to further neutralize exfoliation and infuse water into skin. A Lucas spray could also be utilized.

Active Ingredient Infusion:

Infusion done with a serum that focuses on hydration and antioxidant protection could contain hyaluronic acid, ceramides, and vitamin C. The products purposed should improve the moisture content of the skin, decrease free radicals created by peel, and should be water based.

Mask:

Mask should be a water-based gel with minerals or a collagen sheet mask to enhance hydration and have some occlusion. Minimum application time is 10 minutes, use per manufacturer instructions.

Massage:

The massage medium should be lipid rich, and the massage should incorporate some gentle effleurage movements with some medium-depth movements. The goal is to increase free water in the epidermis by stimulating lymph capillaries and slow TEWL through lipid-based products and increasing microcirculation.

Moisturizing and Protection:

Moisturization should be a water-based cream for oily skin with the use of a lipid barrier enhancement serum (for example, ceramides and sphingolipids) and a broad spectrum (UVA and UVB protection) SPF 15 or higher.

Working with darker Fitzpatrick types or those with impaired healing requires advanced knowledge of the acids available for use and how they affect skin. It is not unusual for a medical esthetician to use a TCA peel on a darker Fitzpatrick type, but the prepping involved is important. The skin must undergo a program of prepping at least six weeks before the actual peel. This can include weekly acid peels, daily application of a retinoid or AHA, a melanin-suppressant product, and sunscreen. Client compliance is mandatory with this type of treatment.

ESTHETIC TECHNOLOGY

The use of technology has been an important part of the professional esthetic treatment for many years. Treating aging skin requires advanced techniques which technology can often provide. To get effective results for an aging client, it is important for an esthetician to understand the options available within his or her scope of practice as well as what technology is available at the medical level. Chapter 7 will cover the basics of technology at the medical level.

Equipment of interest to the esthetician when treating an aging client is as follows:

- Galvanic current
- Ultrasound and machines

ionized solution

ionized solutions are called electrolyte; they are conductors of electricity; ionized solutions are used under the electrodes to facilitate absorption into the epidermis.

positive pole

when galvanic current is introduced into the electrolyte solution, the ions begin to move to either the positive pole, called the anode, or the negative pole, called the cathode.

vasoconstrictive

Constriction of blood vessels.

negative pole

creates an alkaline reaction that is vasodilative; this increases microcirculation, stimulates nerve tissues, causes saponification, and softens tissues.

vasodilative

relaxing or enlarging of blood vessels.

saponification

chemical processes that produce soap from fatty acid derivatives.

iontophoresis

ionized solutions are used under the electrodes to facilitate absorption into the epidermis, a process known as iontophoresis.

electrolytes

ionized solutions are called electrolytes; they are conductors of electricity.

cation

When electrolytes are dissolved in water, they split and form ions that carry either a positive or negative charge. A positively charged ion is a cation.

- Microdermabrasion
- Microcurrent
- Electroporation
- LED light therapy

Galvanic Current

Galvanic therapy is one of the most effective and misunderstood esthetic modalities, even though it has been used for over 70 years in the esthetic industry. It is affordable and easy to use after you understand the basic applications. Galvanic therapy is also used in the medical profession to penetrate various drugs into localized areas of the body.

Functions

Galvanic therapy is used to deep clean the skin, increase absorption of water-soluble products, reduce superficial swelling and puffiness, increase microcirculation in the cells, and improve skin texture (Figure 6–5). It is also used in body treatments for the effect of increased cell metabolism and penetration of products.

How It Works

A direct current is passed through an **ionized solution** into the skin; this solution is water based, which creates a chemical response within the epidermis that can be regulated to target specific nerve endings. The chemical effects caused by galvanic current are used to improve the condition of the skin. Two reactions are created in the skin: under the **positive pole,** an acid reaction is created that is **vasoconstrictive;** it is soothing to nerve endings and firms tissues. The **negative pole** creates an alkaline reaction that is **vasodilative;** this increases microcirculation, stimulates nerve tissues, causes **saponification,** and softens tissues.

Ionized solutions are used under the electrodes to facilitate absorption into the epidermis, a process known as **iontophoresis.** Ionized solutions are called **electrolytes,** and they are conductors of electricity. Electrolytes contain salts and acids, which increase conductivity. When electrolytes are dissolved in water, they split and form ions that carry either a positive or negative charge. A positively charged ion is called a **cation,** and a negatively charged ion is called an **anion.**

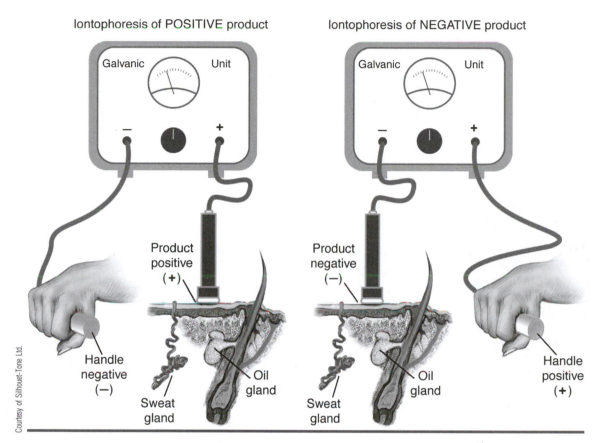

Iontophoresis of POSITIVE product

Iontophoresis of NEGATIVE product

Figure 6–5 An example of a combination machine used for galvanic therapy.

When galvanic current is introduced into the electrolyte solution, the ions begin to move to either the positive pole, called the **anode**, or the negative pole, called the **cathode**. Because the fluids in the body have electrolytic properties, they allow the current to pass through the tissue, thus creating chemical effects in the skin.

Effects of the Positive Pole (Anode)
The effects of the positive pole are:

- Soothing of nerve response
- Constriction of blood vessels

anion

When electrolytes are dissolved in water, they split and form ions that carry either a positive or negative charge. A negatively charged ion is an anion.

anode

When galvanic current is introduced into the electrolyte solution, the ions move to either the positive pole, called the anode, or the negative pole, called the cathode.

cathode
When galvanic current is introduced into the electrolyte solution, the ions move to either the positive pole, called the anode, or the negative pole, called the cathode.

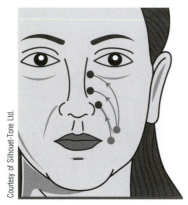

Figure 6–6 Microcurrent machines are used for firming and toning the skin.

- Reduced blood flow
- Tightening and firming of tissues
- Astringent action
- Germicidal action

Effects of the Negative Pole (Cathode)
The effects of the negative pole are:

- Stimulation of nerve response
- Dilation of blood vessels and increased blood flow
- Softening and even desquamation of tissues
- Emulsification and removal of grease (desincrustation)

Microcurrent

Microcurrent is one of the most popular anti-aging technologies used by estheticians. It is used by alternative medicine practitioners for healing injuries, and estheticians use it for firming and toning the skin. Results are reported to be immediate and continue to improve with each subsequent use (Figure 6–6).

Functions

Microcurrent rejuvenates facial muscles, increases cellular functioning, improves skin tone and texture, improves lymphatic circulation, and increases circulation.

How It Works

Microcurrent is micro-amperage stimulation, which is insufficient to activate motor nerves that would cause muscle movement. Microcurrent works with the body's own electrical impulses to increase cellular reactions that slow down as we age, get injured, have an illness, or experience an increase in stress. Microcurrent assists the body by mimicking the body's bioelectric currents. This leads to the repairing of tissue and increased cellular metabolism, activity, and exchange.

Microcurrent uses direct electric currents ranging from 10 mA to 500 mA at varied waveforms and frequencies. Some manufacturers include a faradic current, which is an interrupted AC current. Technology is rapidly changing; a new addition to the microcurrent market is the use of nanotechnology. The theory is that nanocurrent, current in the range of one-billionth of an ampere, is more readily recognized by the cells; these currents have been shown to even produce amperage in the pico range, or one-trillionth of an ampere.

Most manufacturers have their own proprietary information about how their machines produce currents and waveforms. The different waveforms used are *square, sine, rectangle,* and *pulsed.* These are standard waveforms recognized within electrical engineering; how a company chooses to modify and market them is the key to selling their machines. Also used are low- and high-frequency currents that also are proprietary to certain manufacturers.

When direct microcurrent is used, it affects more than just the skin tissue: the correct movements that the esthetician uses will also lengthen or shorten various muscle groups. It is important to understand the muscles of the face and where the insertion and origin of each muscle is. For example, to firm the nasolabial folds, you would shorten the muscle with a specific movement.

Microcurrent will reprogram the muscle fiber, allowing it to be lengthened or shortened, depending on the direction of the application. When a muscle contracts and shortens, one of its attachments usually remains fixed, and the other one moves.

The Effects of Microcurrent

Microcurrent causes multiple effects in the skin and body:

- **Increases ATP:** This molecule is involved in the cell to provide cellular energy transport and enzyme regulation. A study done by Cheng and colleagues (1982)[2] reported that microcurrent increased ATP as much as 500 percent. When ATP metabolism is reduced in the cell, the aging process is accelerated, and the signs of aging appear at a faster rate.
- **Increases fibroblast activity:** Fibroblast cells are large oval cells found in connective tissue. They are responsible for producing collagen and elastin in the skin. Collagen and elastin are some of the most important parts of our skin; when we age, they deteriorate and cause a loss of firmness.
- **Increases protein synthesis:** Muscles are largely influenced by proteins that also act as part of antioxidant defenses. Elastin and collagen are also proteins.
- **Increases cell permeability:** When the body ages, cells become less permeable, so various functions in the body slow down. Transepidermal water loss (TEWL) is reduced by microcurrent, so the skin stays hydrated, which creates the correct pH for **homeostasis**

homeostasis
the maintenance of normal, internal stability in the body.

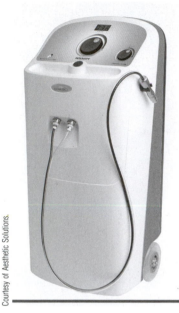

Courtesy of Aesthetic Solutions.

Figure 6–7 Microder-
mabrasion machines are
used to treat rhytids,
dyschromia,
hyperpigmentation,
and keratinized skin.

rhytids
wrinkles.

dyschromia
disorder of pigmentation in skin and
hair.

hyperpigmentation
over production of melanin resulting
from UVR ultraviolet radiation, or injury.

keratin (keratinized)
skin cells with no nucleous found in the
stratum corneum.

in the skin. This is important in order for the cells to absorb more nutrients, oxygen, and water; it also helps the cells excrete toxins to the lymph system and blood system.

Microdermabrasion

Microdermabrasion is one of most effective treatment modalities that an esthetician can use today. It is a simple technology with clinical studies to prove its efficacy. It requires adequate training to provide optimal benefits. It is an operator-dependent technology, which means that outcomes can be different with each operator (Figure 6–7). It is wonderful for the treatment of **rhytids**, **dyschromia**, **hyperpigmentation,** and **keratinized** skin.

How It Works

A vacuum is created by a compressor that draws air from the atmosphere when the hand piece is applied to the skin. This causes the aluminum oxide crystals to be moved by negative pressure to the hand piece, which then flows to the surface of the skin, causing exfoliation, the epidermal debris and crystals are returned via a separate tube to a disposal canister or filter bag. The depth of exfoliation is controlled by vacuum and crystal flow.

The other popular alternative is the diamond-encrusted tip, which uses the same vacuum technology but has no crystals flowing through the system. It provides exfoliation by moving different hand pieces with various diamond grit types over the surface of the skin.

Effects of Microdermabrasion

Microdermabrasion causes the following effects:

- Increased desquamation of the skin due to the exfoliation of the stratum corneum, which will smooth coarse skin, soften fine lines and wrinkles, decrease the appearance of scarring and pore size, and reduce superficial hyperpigmentation.
- Increased microcirculation in the skin, which will improve the transport of oxygen and nutrients to the cells.
- With multiple uses, theorized to stimulate cellular functions of the dermal and epidermal layers, which can cause an increase in collagen production.
- Increased lymphatic drainage, which reduces puffiness and eliminates accumulated wastes.

LED Light Therapy

LED light therapy is also known as photo rejuvenation, and photo therapy. LED light therapy is considered a non-laser light source and is available to estheticians. It is primarily being used for anti-aging treatments and more currently acne treatments.

LED is considered a low power, non-thermal light device, unlike lasers, which use high power coherent light (Figure 6–8). LED light therapy uses non-coherent light in various wavelengths, generally in the red, infrared, and blue spectrums. Light therapy remains controversial within the medical and scientific community. Not many studies are run for widely accepted peer review journals. We will take a look at the widely accepted functions of LED light therapy for the beauty industry with the understanding that they have not been scientifically proven, but observations within the esthetic community support the assumptions.

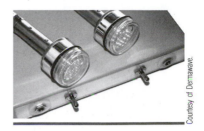

Figure 6–8 LED light therapy is considered a non-laser light source available to estheticians.

How It Works

A machine produces non-coherent light in a specific color or wavelength, specific strength or joules, with multiple frequencies, using light-emitting diodes applied by handheld probes in a pattern or by a face plate placed about an inch from the face for certain length of time.

The electrical components of the light are encased by a clear epoxy with a metallurgy compound coated over the electrical junction of the LED light bulb. These compounds are known as inorganic semiconductor materials. When excited by an electrical voltage, particular colors are emitted. See Figure 6–9 for a chart of inorganic semiconductor materials used.

Different colors, such as red and blue, are used to activate different cellular responses in the skin, much like a plant grows under the sun. The greatest cellular reaction happens closest to the light source.

Effects of Red light 624 nm, 630 nm–680 nm, and Infrared Light 950 nm:

Many machines produce red light at 624 nm, 633 nm, and 660 nm; each is considered the optimal wavelength for the following:

- Increases circulation: speeds up the healing process by supplying additional oxygen and nutrients to the cell.
- Stimulates collagen production: collagen is an essential protein that holds cells together and gives firmness to the skin.
- Stimulates ATP: adenosine triphosphate is the major carrier of energy to all cells. It increases the energy level of cells, which

Semiconductor Materials	Color Wavelength Created
AigAaS	Red and infrared
AlGaP	Green
AlGaInP	High bright orange, red, yellow, green
GaAsP	Red, orange-red, orange, yellow
GaP – gallium phosphide	Red, yellow, green
GaN	Green, emerald green, blue
InGaN	Near ultraviolet, blue green, blue
SiC – silicon carbide	Blue
Si – silicon	Blue
$A_{12}O_3$ – sapphire	Blue
ZnSe – zinc selenide	Blue
C – diamond	Ultraviolet
AlN – aluminium nitride	Near to far ultraviolet
AlGaN	Near to far ultraviolet
AlGaInN	Near to far ultraviolet

Figure 6–9 Chart of inorganic semiconductors.

leads to increased cell production. One theory of aging is that the ability for cells to produce energy is reduced, which leads to many symptoms of aging.

- Increases lymphatic flow.
- Increases RNA and DNA synthesis: damaged cells are replaced more quickly.
- Stimulates fibroblastic activity: aids in the repair process, helps form collagen.
- Increases phagocytosis: a process of finding and ingesting dead or dying cells by the phagocyte cells. This will help reduce inflammation.
- Increases thermal effect: it will increase the temperature of the cells, without heating the surface of the skin. This may lead to better product penetration.

Color	Effect
Red	Increased circulation, stimulation of fibroblasts, stimulation of ATP, increased lymphatic flow, increased cell rejuvenation and metabolism
Amber	Same effects as red when used at 590 nm
Yellow	Increased lymphatic flow
Green	Decreased melanin production
Blue	Kills *P. acnes* bacteria
Infrared	Increased circulation and heat in tissues, which helps with pain relief

© Milady, a part of Cengage Learning.

Figure 6–10 Chart of LED colors and their effects.

Effects of Blue Light 415 nm–480 nm

This wavelength was recently studied as a treatment for acne. The finding was that blue light at 415 nm and red light at 660 nm are more effective than blue light alone.[3]

This produces singlet oxygen, which kills the *P. acnes* bacteria (*Propionibacterium acnes*).

Effects of Yellow

Yellow light at 590 nm is used for its healing, draining, and detoxifying properties. It is absorbed by the body fluids in the lymph and blood circulatory systems and promotes wound healing. It increases lymphatic flow to evacuate more waste products and boosts cellular activity.

Effects of Green

Green light at 525 nm decreases melanin production, reduces pigmentation, and eliminates the redness associated with the use of chemical peel and bleaching products.

See Figure 6–10 chart of colors and their biological effect.

Ultrasound and Low Frequency Ultrasound Machines

Ultrasound is one of the more recent modalities introduced into the esthetics industry, and it is controversial. Physical therapists and other allied health professionals usually use therapeutic ultrasound for pain

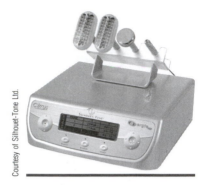

Courtesy of Silhouet-Tone Ltd.

Figure 6–11 Ultrasound machines work by using sound waves at specific frequencies to create physical changes at the cellular level.

piezoelectric effect
electrical charge created when the crystal is subjected to mechanical pressure.

management and for healing injury. This equipment is considered a Class II prescriptive device, which means it must come with a label (Figure 6–11). Many states consider this device outside the scope of esthetics practice, and it may be hard to get liability insurance to cover its use, because it can cause harm to the body if not used correctly. But it has also shown promising results in the care of aging skin.

Low frequency ultrasound has been recently introduced into the esthetic market with interesting studies supporting safe outcomes for transdermal transport. Low frequency ultrasound uses ultrasound waves at 20 KHz, instead of the 3 MHz that is usually used in the esthetic and medical professions. Research has shown that low frequency ultrasound did not produce damage to the barrier function or damage to living cells.[4] The mechanism used for transdermal absorption is still cavitations, but the effects are on the outside as well as the inside of the stratum corneum. This has been hypothesized to create channels within the lipid bilayers in which larger molecules can pass. This is seen in the therapeutic application of sonophoresis as well, except the delivery of the active ingredients is more effective.

How It Works

Ultrasound works by using sound waves at specific frequencies to create physical changes at the cellular level. The frequencies are measured in megahertz (MHz), and ultrasound works at a range exceeding 20,000 cycles per second.

Ultrasound energy is created by a crystal contained in the sound head; the crystal converts normal 10-volt energy from the outlet using a transformer. The conversion of energy to ultrasound occurs through a scientific principle called the **piezoelectric effect**. This is when an electrical charge is delivered to the crystal that creates mechanical pressure, which causes the crystal to vibrate and produce sound waves.

The ultrasonic waves are delivered through tissue via a coupling medium. This medium is a specifically created glycerin or water-based gel that allows the ultrasound energy to pass through it. The tissue density also effects how the ultrasound is delivered into the tissue. Tissue with the highest protein content will absorb most effectively.

Therapeutic ultrasound has a frequency range of 1 MHz to 3 MHz. The lower the frequency, the deeper it penetrates. For example, 1 MHz can penetrate bone. This is not to be confused with the commonly called *ultrasonic machine,* which creates high frequency mechanical oscillations in the range of 25,000 to 28,000 vibrations per second. This ultrasonic machine uses a metal spatula to exfoliate the skin in a process called **cavitation,** which creates bubbles in water or an ultrasound gel that implodes when the ultrasound energy creates compression and refraction in the medium. Unstable cavitation places stress on thinner structures, which could cause rupture and cell or tissue destruction. Unstable cavitation occurs when the bubbles created by sound waves explode under pressure. This can be caused by continuous high frequency ultrasound application.

Effects of Ultrasound/Ultrasonic Machines

Therapeutic ultrasound for esthetic purposes primarily uses sonophoresis, which is a means of penetrating a special ultrasonic gel with active ingredients deep into the skin. This process is most beneficial at a range of 20 to 25 KHz with the waveform pulsed on and off every second. This is also the method for low frequency ultrasound transdermal penetration. **Sonophoresis** is effective at creating microscopic channels, called **lacunae,** in the intercellular layers of the skin. This opens up the intercellular pathways that allow products with a high molecular weight a better degree of penetration.

Therapeutic ultrasound also has the following benefits:

- Increases temperature within the skin, which stimulates circulation, lymph drainage, and cell metabolism
- Increases cell permeability
- Increases intracellular calcium, a messenger for cell function
- Helps speed up the inflammatory healing response

Electroporation

Electroporation is relatively new in the esthetic industry. It is like sonophoresis except that electroporation creates aqueous channels directly into the cellular structure through electric pulses applied directly to the skin. It is used for transdermal drug delivery and chemotherapy enhancement as well as in molecular biology to transform DNA.

How It Works

The lipid bilayer around the cell's membrane has a hydrophilic exterior and a hydrophobic interior. This means that DNA, proteins, and any polar molecules are unable to pass through the membrane. Electroporation provides short electrical pulses within milliseconds at 100 volts or less, which essentially punches holes within the lipid bilayer. This allows molecules to pass, and then the lipid bilayer quickly repairs itself and seals the molecule within the cell interior.

cavitation
formation and collapse of bubbles in a liquid by means of a mechanical force.

sonophoresis
action caused by low level ultrasound which is used to penetrate active ingredients through channels called lacunae.

lacunae
See *sonophoresis*.

The Effects of Electroporation

The effects of electroporation on the skin have been studied primarily in drug delivery studies. The concern is that *in vivo* studies have shown that cell death can occur when the voltage is the wrong strength or intensity due to the holes failing to close after application. The main effect of electroporation is delivery of active ingredients into the cellular structure of the skin, which would be wholly dependent on the type of ingredients being delivered. This modality has been seen in the esthetic industry as part of multi-modality equipment.

Layering Modalities and Multiple-use Machines

One technology by itself may not be enough to address the complex nature of aging skin. Many manufacturers have created new machines that combine multiple technologies to address aging from a muscle, dermal, and epidermal standpoint. The challenge for the esthetician is determining safety as well as scope-of-practice issues. Everything that is done at an esthetic level indirectly affects all of the layers of the skin as well as impacting the entire body.

The challenge comes when the modality used changes the structure of the skin. In the future many licensing agencies will need to look at the difference between temporary structure changes and permanent changes such as those seen with an aesthetic medical modality.

The use of multiple modalities and layering technology is one of the most efficient and successful treatment practices that an esthetician can employ. For example, combining microdermabrasion with iontophoresis for penetration of a product to treat hyperpigmentation is effective. Another helpful option is layering microcurrent with microdermabrasion. Microdermabrasion done first will allow the active ingredients to penetrate more easily when microcurrent is applied. Figure 6–12 represents an example of multi-function anti-aging equipment.

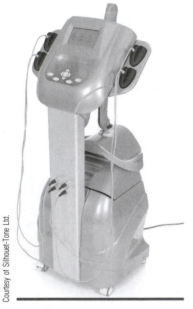

Courtesy of Silhouet-Tone Ltd.

Figure 6–12 Silhouet-Tone Skin Remodeling System rejuvenation machine is one example of multi-function anti-aging equipment.

▪ HEALTHY AGING MAKEUP

Makeup is one of the most effective and often overlooked modalities that can provide an immediate benefit to the client if applied correctly. Aging clients can have many physical challenges when using makeup, such as:

- Poor mobility due to arthritis, fibromyalgia, injuries
- Poor eyesight
- Finding skin-type-appropriate makeup
- Getting accurate, unbiased information
- Knowing how to correctly take care of their skin

- Finding a professional who understands issues and has technical knowledge

The solutions to these challenges are varied but can include:

- For poor eyesight, provide a magnifying mirror
- Large-handled makeup brushes
- Easy application techniques
- Lash extensions
- Lash and brow tinting
- Teaching and communicating clearly
- Active listening
- Providing tools for home use

All estheticians have basic makeup knowledge through their professional training; however, these additional techniques can help address the specific needs of the aging client.

Foundation and Contouring

Choosing a foundation should be based on skin type, skin undertone, color, depth, and type of coverage needed. The color should match the neck and should have a soft dewy finish. Foundation is most effective when applied with a makeup sponge or foundation brush depending on formulation type. A stripe test is always needed when deciding on the correct color.

Techniques

To Make the Face Look Thinner:

After foundation application, use a powder contour color two to three shades darker than skin tone. Blend well at jaw line and under cheekbones. Use a highlight color at the upper part of cheekbones (see Figure 6–13 for an example).

To Reduce the Appearance of Wrinkles:

Apply a primer then liquid foundation with a dewy or soft finish. Set with a translucent matte powder. Then use a small face brush and place a matte highlight color, which is one to two shades lighter than the skin tone, inside of the wrinkle. Gently blend.

To Thin the Nose:

After foundation application, apply contour powder one shade darker along the outer portion of nose, and a lighter highlight color to the bridge of the nose and inner corner of eyes (Figure 6–14).

A stripe test consists of applying two or three shades along jaw line to neck, then waiting a minute to see how the color adjusts to the skin. For darker skin tones or skin with hyperpigmentation, use a stripe from the cheek to jaw line. In some cases two colors of foundation may be needed.

Dark colors recede areas they are applied to; light colors bring out areas they are applied to. Remember to balance both when trying to create a contour illusion.

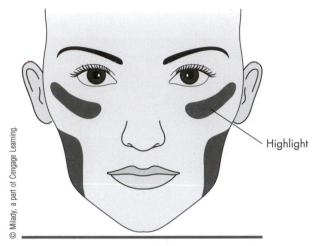

Figure 6–13 Face contour placement.

To Reduce Double Chin:

After foundation application, apply contour powder from edge to underneath the jaw line. Blend well. Apply highlight color and matte finish to the center of the chin (Figure 6–15).

Cover hyperpigmentation and **telangiectasia**: Before applying foundation, apply with concealer brush a cream concealer directly on the pigmented spot or broken vein. Do not apply outside of area being covered. Use your finger to stipple (gently pat) edges around area being covered. Apply foundation in stipple fashion in order to

telengiectasia
couperose, or broken capillaries.

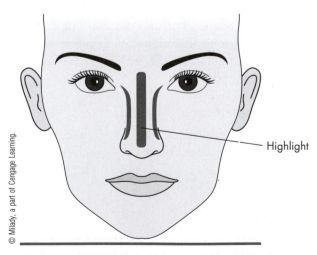

Figure 6–14 Nose contour placement.

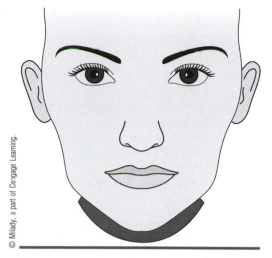

Figure 6–15 Double chin contour placement.

avoid removing the concealer, and then apply powder to set. If using mineral makeup, use a large soft brush and gently blend.

Eye Techniques

Eyes are one of the first areas of the face to show aging and are one of the areas that many clients have a hard time using makeup on. Techniques that are used in magazines are usually too harsh for the aging client. Some simple color and technique changes could take years off (Figure 6–16).

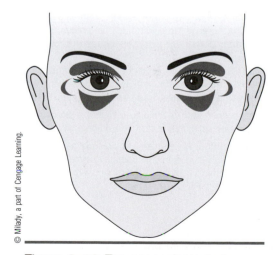

Figure 6–16 Eye concealer technique.

Note: this client has multiple skin conditions that will take a series of progressive treatments to improve. Start with immediate hydration, exfoliation, and infusion of active ingredients.

Over-hydrating skin during a facial is a good rule of thumb. Always do more than the client will at home. For example: serum, moisturizer, and sunscreen.

Client Example

Now let's look at our case study:

Client: 42-year-old female

Skin type: Combination–Fitzpatrick Type 2

Conditions: Photodamage (hyperpigmentation), fine lines, (stage 1 aging), dehydration, hyperkeratinized (dead skin cell buildup), comedones (blackheads)

Assessment: Client has identified with wrong skin type thus using the wrong home care products, high stress levels are impacting hydration and texture issues in the skin. Perimenopausal symptoms are adding to skin condition. Fitzpatrick type is good for most clinical treatments.

Goal: Increase desquamation to reduce fine lines, increase fibroblast stimulation, hydration (free water in the epidermis), increase microcirculation and lymphatic flow (oxygenation of the skin), exfoliate the stratum corneum, suppress melanin production (inhibit tyrosinase production, reduce melanosome transfer), reduce inflammation, increase free radical protection, and induce the relaxation response in the body.

- Even if hyperpigmentation is the client's primary concern, the skin must have good hydration and a repaired barrier before treating pigmentation issues. This is where understanding the function of each layer of skin is important so that the client can be educated about the process.

Based on these goals and the purpose of each, phase one of the treatments would look like this:

Stimulation Phase Goals–Cleansing: first cleansing done with a makeup remover or gel cleanser. Second cleanse done with a gel cleanser created for combination skin.

Toning: toning phase is done with a pH balancing, hydrating toner.

Exfoliation: proteolytic enzyme mask with steam.

Toning: toning phase is done with gentle hydrating toner to further neutralize exfoliation and infuse water into skin.

Active Ingredient Infusion: infusion done with a serum.

Massage: The massage medium should be lipid rich, and the massage should incorporate some gentle effleurage movements with some medium-depth movements. The goal is to increase free water in the epidermis by stimulating lymph capillaries and slow TEWL through lipid-based products and increasing microcirculation.

Mask: Mask should be designed to enhance hydration and have some occlusion; a firming compression mask to stimulate lymph movement would be beneficial. Minimum application time 10 minutes, use per manufacturer instructions.

Toning: toning phase done with a tonic to infuse the skin with active ingredients. Antioxidants, peptides, or anti-inflammatory ingredients would be helpful.

Moisturizing and Protection: Moisturizer should be a balanced humectant or emollient blend for combination skin with the use of a melanin-suppressant serum (for example, kojic acid, vitamin C, alpha arbutin) applied first and a broad spectrum (UVA and UVB protection) SPF 30 or higher.

- **Puffy eyes**: Apply eye cream, foundation. Then with a small eye brush or highlighting pen, apply in the crease just underneath puffiness. If concealing dark circles as well, apply concealer to area of discoloration and then highlight. Set with a soft translucent powder.
- **Dark circles**: Apply before foundation with a concealer brush and a cream concealer, close to skin tone. On only the area of darkness, gently stipple with your finger around edges to blend in. Apply foundation and set with translucent finishing powder.
- **Sparse lashes**: Curl lashes, then apply lash primer. Use mascara formulation with small brush starting at base of lashes and gently moving outward. There are many mascara formulations that claim to build lashes, but avoid anything that contains fibers. Focus on lash length rather than thickness. Thick, clumpy lashes can make the eyes look older. Lash extensions and small clusters of false lashes are also techniques that can be used.

> A yellow-based concealer is best for light skin tones, and a golden-orange tone is better for darker skin tones. Ebony skin can use a warm-brown tone.

▶ ▷ ▷ Top Ten Tips to Take to the Clinic

1. When designing a treatment, focus on the client's primary concerns while keeping in mind the physiology of the skin.
2. It is important to understand the purpose of each step in the facial treatment.
3. Utilize technology to accelerate results.
4. Master massage techniques such as manual lymph drainage (MLD) and facelift massage movements.
5. Understand the goal, visual signs, and options for treatment when determining what to incorporate in a facial treatment.
6. Layering modalities is an effective way to get accelerated results.
7. Correct makeup color can make the skin look younger.
8. Contouring can be used to reduce a sagging jaw line.
9. Dark colors make the areas they cover recede; light colors bring out the areas they cover.
10. Thick, clumpy lashes make the eyes look older.

Chapter Review Questions

1. What is the purpose of the cleansing phase?
2. What is the purpose of the exfoliation phase?
3. What is the purpose of the active infusion phase?
4. What benefits does massage provide the skin?
5. What types of exfoliation are good for hyperpigmentation?

References

1. Lees, M. (2001). *Skin Care: Beyond the Basics*. Clifton Park, NY: Thomson Delmar Learning.
2. Baumann, L. MD., Saghari, S. MD., Weisburg, E. MS. (2009). *Cosmetic Dermatology; Principles and Practice*, 2nd Edition. New York: McGraw Hill Medical.
3. Nordman, L. (2005). *Professional Beauty Therapy: The Official Guide to Level*, 2nd Ed. London: Thomson Learning.
4. Mitragotri, S., Blankschtein, D., Langer, R. (1996). "Transdermal Drug Delivery Using Low Frequency Sonophoresis." *Pharmaceutical Research:* Vol. 13, No. 3., NY: Kluwer Academic/Plenum Publishers.

Bibliography

Prausnitiz, M.R., et al. (1993). "Electroporation of Mammalian Skin: A Mechanism to Enhance Transdermal Drug Delivery." *National Academy of Sciences:* Vol. 90, 10504–10508.

Schmaling, S. (2008). *Milady's Aesthetician Series: A Comprehensive Guide to Equipment*. Clifton Park, NY: Milady, a part of Cengage Learning.

Culp, J., et al. (2010). *Milady's Standard Esthetics: Advanced*, 1st Edition. Clifton Park, NY: Milady Cengage Learning.

Jones, R. (2008). *Looking Younger: Makeovers That Make You Look as Young as You Feel*. Beverly, MA: Fair Winds Press.

Barrett-Hill, F. (2010). *Cosmetic Chemistry*. Whangaparoa, New Zealand: Virtual Beauty Corporation Ltd.

Websites

Massage Education:
www.belavi.com
www.naturestones.com
www.upledger.com
www.faceliftmassage.com

Professional Products

Chapter 7

Key Terms

cosmeceuticals
hydrophilic
inert

International
Nomenclature of
Cosmetic
Ingredients
(INCI)

microorganisms
phospholipids
vesicles

Learning Objectives

After completing this chapter, you will be able to:

1. Explain the basics of cosmetic chemistry.
2. Describe the different categories of professional products.
3. Recognize the basics of key ingredients.
4. Identify the key ingredients that can cause harm.

■ INTRODUCTION

Clients are always asking what the difference is between products bought at drugstores and the professional products offered by the esthetician. Choosing the correct professional products for the treatment of aging skin is one of the most common challenges an esthetician will face. The line between *professional* and *mass market* is getting thinner, and clients are more ingredient savvy than ever. The anti-aging market is a multibillion-dollar industry with no slowdown in sight; therefore the competition between product lines is fierce.

How does an esthetician sort through the marketing hype to make a science-based decision? It requires a basic understanding of the physiology of the skin, cosmetic chemistry, and a healthy dose of critical thinking. Throughout this chapter we will be looking at the most effective known ingredients to treat aging skin. This is a short listing of the exciting ingredients available to estheticians. The esthetician should pursue this area of study through advanced education classes and books.

■ COSMETIC CHEMISTRY BASICS

The basics of cosmetic chemistry are covered in the basic esthetic training required for licensing. Rather than go through the basic information again, let's take a different approach and focus on the purpose of many cosmetic formulations. The FDA defines cosmetics as follows:

- Articles intended to be rubbed, poured, sprinkled, or sprayed on, introduced into, or otherwise applied to the human body or any part thereof for cleansing, beautifying, promoting attractiveness, or altering the appearance, and articles intended for use as a component of any such articles; except that such term shall not include soap.[1]

This definition corresponds with the scope-of-practice guidelines that most states have for esthetician licensing. This is a broad description which leaves substantial wiggle room for manufacturers to create products that can be considered drugs if some of their claims were investigated. Because of the advances in the cosmetic chemistry industry in the field of more active and reparative ingredients, a new category was coined in the 1990s by Dr. Albert Kligman called **cosmeceuticals**. This category has not been recognized by the FDA but is regularly used in the profession.

The reality is that most formulations are designed only to enhance the skin's surface and provide basic protection. The real focus from a professional esthetic formulation point of view is to create products that

cosmeceuticals
a term coined by Dr. Albert Kligman to describe topical cosmetics that are designed to improve the appearance of the skin through delivery of active ingredients into the epidermis.

mimic the skin's own protective barrier, support the skin functions, and treat specific issues.

Often the first thing that an esthetician looks at is the ingredient in a product to see if it works for them. The important thing to remember is that it is the formulation that makes the difference. The formulation of a product will stabilize and ensure the correct dosage of the active ingredients, allow for better delivery, and make it safe for use. There are basic categories of formulations and ingredients, and each has a specific purpose, as outlined in the sections that follow.

Ingredients

There are basic categories of ingredients.

Skin Conditioning Ingredients:
The focus is to improve the stratum corneum using emollients and humectants.

Performance Ingredients:
Used to treat specific skin conditions, can be unstable and usually need a delivery system to get the actives into the skin. Correct formulation and dosage will determine the effectiveness. Examples are retinol, vitamin C, and peptides. Also known as active ingredients.

Functional Ingredients:
Used to stabilize the formulation and mix together ingredients such as those outlined in the sections that follow.

Emulsion: A liquid that joins two or more unmixable ingredients together through an emulsifier. An emulsion helps oil penetrate the skin, which slows TEWL. They are classified as:

- Oil in water (o/w) emulsion (most common formulations)
- Water in oil (w/o) emulsion
- Water in silicone (w/si) emulsion

Surfactant: An ingredient that reduces the surface tension of fluids. See Table 7–1 for a chart of common surfactants. Surfactants are used in the following:

- Cleansers—used as detergents
- Creams and lotions—used as emulsifiers
- Hair care products—used as conditioning agents and wetting agents
- Perfumes—used as solubilizers

When looking at cosmetic ingredients, you will often notice two names. One is this organization: **International Nomenclature of Cosmetic Ingredients (INCI).** This listing is a system of names for cosmetic ingredients used internationally by chemists and regulators. The second name is the trade name that the ingredient is sold under, which is common with engineered cosmetic ingredient formulations.

International Nomenclature of Cosmetic Ingredients (INCI) a stanardized system of names for chemicals used in cosmetics, required by regulatory agencies and chemists.

Table 7–1 Chart of nonionic and biosurfactants.

Type of Surfactant	Name of Ingredient	Actions
Anionic	Sodium lauryl sulfate Sodium dodecyl sulfate Ammonium lauryl sulfate Sodium laureth sulfate Alkyl benzene sulfonate	High foaming, most commonly used emulsifier, stable, can be irritating, inexpensive
Amphoteric	Disodium cocoamphodipropionate Disodium cocoamphodiacetate Sodium cocoamphoacetate Sodium cocoamphopropionate	Mild action, used in formulas to lessen effects of harsh surfactants
Nonionic	Fatty alcohols–cetyl/oleyl Ethylene oxide Octyl glucoside n-Dodecyl-beta-D-Maltoside Cocamide MEA, DEA Polysorbates Glyceryl esters–glycerin Glyceryl monostearates	Low reactivity, safe
Cationic	Ammonium lauryl sulfate Dodecyl trimethylammonium Cetyl trimethylammonium bromide Cetylpyridinium chloride Benzalkonium chloride Benzethonium chloride	High reactivity, irritating, should not be used in professional skin care products

© Milady, a part of Cengage Learning.

Thickeners: These ingredients increase viscosity, stabilize suspensions, and create an aesthetically appealing feel. Some common thickeners are:

- Seaweeds—carrageen, alginates
- Beeswax
- Xanthan gum
- Paraffin
- Cetyl alcohol

Preservatives: These ingredients retard **microorganisms** and fungus growth, and bind metal ions and stop their reactivity (chelate), which is important for the stability of the product and prevention of infection. Usually a synthetic ingredient is used for safety, but there are also some natural preservatives that require special airless packaging and have a short shelf life (Table 7–2).

Some commonly used preservatives are outlined in the sections that follow.

Multi-functional Ingredients: These ingredients provide functional benefits as well as assist the delivery system to get active ingredients in the skin. Some examples are:

- Sorbitol
- Cetyl alcohol
- Glycol stearate

Preservatives are always a controversial issue. The only way a product can be truly preservative free is to have a low pH and high percentage of alcohol. Some unethical *preservative-free* claims come from the fact that the manufacturer will list only one function of a multi-functional ingredient.

microorganisms
microscopic forms of life such as gram positive and negative bacteria; yeast.and fungus

Table 7–2 Most common preservative groups.

Common Preservatives	Concerns and Source
Parabens	Concerns about estrogenic activity
DMDM hydantoin	Formaldehyde releaser–most commonly used in cosmetics
Quaternium-15	Formaldehyde releaser–banned in Japan and Sweden, major cause of dermatitis
Imidazolidinyl urea	Formaldehyde releaser
Disodium edetate	No reported issues
Tetrasodium EDTA	Chelating agent
Sodium benzoate	No reported issues
Methylisothiazolinone	Used in preservative blends
Phenoxyethanol	Used in preservative blends
Benzalkonium chloride	Can be irritating
Grapefruit seed extract–60%	Natural source, somewhat unstable, no long shelf life
Tea tree	Natural source, cannot be used as a preservative by itself, toxic in high percentages
Citric acid	Natural source, chelating agent

inert
will not react with other ingredients.

Solvents: Clear, colorless liquids used to help evenly distribute ingredients, reduce viscosity within a formulation and are considered **inert**. Common examples are:

- Water
- SD alcohol
- Isopropyl myristate
- Quaternium-26

Formulations:

The formulation is a combination of various ingredients used together to provide a specific function. They include products outlined in the following sections.

Essential Products:
Essential products are used to maintain healthy skin:

- Lotions, creams, and oils that assist humectants to bind water to the skin. They form a seal so that TEWL will not happen as quickly.
- Cleansers that remove debris and dirt from skin.
- Toners that hydrate and rebalance pH.
- Sunscreen that protects from UV radiation.

Performance Products:
Performance products are used to treat skin conditions:

- Serums used to treat certain skin conditions including the signs of aging.
- Treatment creams formulated to be multi-functional with active ingredients as well as humectants and emollients.
- Masks used for improvement of the stratum corneum and in professional treatments.

Skin Penetration of Products

This is a question often asked by estheticians and clients alike. The benefits of many of the listed ingredients are not effective unless they reach deeply into the epidermis and have an effect on cells. Impacting the cells of the skin often depends on the delivery system used by the manufacturer. Here are some basic absorption facts:

- Absorption is directly affected by the concentration of the substance and the area over which it is applied. For example, lidocaine applied to small areas of the skin is safe; however, applied to large areas, such as legs (especially with occlusion), it can lead to overdose.
- The thickness of the stratum corneum determines the degree of absorption. Areas where this layer of skin is thin, such as the genitals, are much more receptive to absorption than the soles of the feet, where this layer is thicker.

A basic daily skin routine for healthy skin generally is the following:

AM: Goal—hydrate and protect

Cleanse

Tone

Serum

Moisturizer and sun protection

PM: Goal—hydrate and
     rejuvenate

Cleanse

Tone

Serum

Treatment cream

- A damaged skin barrier will facilitate absorption at a faster rate. This is why estheticians should always exfoliate before applying serums and massage; this is also why the lipid barrier is removed before performing a chemical peel.
- Occlusion of the skin enhances product penetration. Occlusion means applying a substance to the skin where air cannot penetrate. You can purchase specific plastic masks that create an occlusive environment in the skin.
- The composition of the product affects its penetration. No one ingredient makes the difference, but rather the molecular weight and how the ingredient is carried. If the ingredient carrier damages the lipid barrier, then absorption will occur at a faster rate.
- Lipid-soluble products will absorb better than others. Any product that is similar to the intercellular *cement* will be readily accepted by the stratum corneum. Below the stratum corneum, the epidermis is **hydrophilic**. The challenge is to find a carrier that will benefit the lipophilic stratum corneum and also the hydrophilic epidermis.
- Increasing the temperature of the skin aids absorption. For this reason, steam can indirectly affect how a product is absorbed: warmer skin will generally absorb products at a faster rate.

hydrophilic
attracted to water molecules.

Ingredient Carriers

Ingredient carriers can be one of the most important parts of an anti-aging formulation. By getting active ingredients to the deeper layers of the epidermis, for example to the dermal-epidermal junction, cells can be influenced to do a variety of things based on the ingredient being presented.

An active ingredient works only if it is accepted by the cell it is trying to target. Most are far too large to penetrate the skin effectively without help. There are additional benefits to a delivery system besides getting the ingredient to the cell; some delivery systems will help protect antioxidants from oxidation and discolorations. Some of the benefits of a delivery system are:

- Prevention of oxidation
- Lengthening of shelf life
- Improving the texture and appearance of a product
- Reduction of irritancy
- Delivering time-released activity
- Helping to combine incompatible ingredients, for example, oil and water

Controlled release is one of the delivery systems that professional products use. This system is used in many different ways, the most common to use ingredients that mimic the skin's lipids in order to *piggyback* active ingredients into the skin. Liposomes are the best example of this.[2]

Liposomes

Liposomes are one of the first carriers designed and are among the most effective. Liposomes are microscopic spheres that are made of layers of phospholipids. **Phospholipids** are lipids that make up the cell membrane. Soybean lecithin phospholipids are the most compatible to the cell membrane, bilayers, and acid mantle. Liposomes also help slow TEWL or transepidermal water loss. Liposomes come in three basic types:[3]

- Small unilamellar **vesicles**
- Large unilamellar vesicles
- Multi-lamellar vesicle structure

How Liposomes Deliver Active Ingredients

Clients frequently ask how products penetrate and work on the skin. This basic theory on how liposomes penetrate could be applied to other delivery systems as well.

1. The formulation is applied to the skin, and the outer shell of the delivery system binds to the keratin of the keratinocyte.
2. The delivery system begins to travel through the lipid bilayers; phospholipids are accepted by the bilayers while the water portion of the formulation is delivered into the stratum corneum.
3. The active ingredients are released as the delivery system melts into the layers of the epidermis and travels to the deeper layers of the skin.[4]

▪ NANOTECHNOLOGY

Nanotechnology has been used for over 20 years for many applications and has no globally recognized definition. The term is assumed to apply to any structure less than 100 nanometers in size. The concerns reside with the concept of potential toxicity with ingredients passing through the skin's barrier into the body.

Nanosomes are the most common form of nanotechnology used within the skin care industry and are similar in makeup to liposomes. They are small single or double bilayer liposomes in a nano size, which is usually around 50 nanometers.[5]

Many nanosomes are created with high quality phospholipids and contain approximately 40 percent phosphatidylcholine, which is an essential component of cell membranes. The processing of nanosomes is complex and expensive, which reflects in the price of the product.

Phospholipids
lipids that are part of the cell membrane.

vesicles
small sac containing fluid.

A nanosome is 800 times smaller than a human hair and approximately 20 times smaller than a liposome.

▪ ESSENTIAL PRODUCTS

Cleansers

Cleansers are one of the most important products to use when trying to improve the skin, and one of the most overlooked by clients. The effects of an acid mantle impaired by cleansing with a high alkaline, low quality surfactant cleansing agent can include the following:

- Damage to the stratum corneum proteins; water used in cleansing is absorbed by the corneocytes and results in protein swelling; surfactants increase the swelling; the amount is determined by the surfactant and pH of the cleanser. Stratum corneum swelling has been shown to increase irritancy and remove the NMF (natural moisture factor) in the skin.[6]
- Damage to the SC lipids and increase in TEWL (transepidermal water loss); surfactants and high pH induce a change in lipid bilayer composition and even partial removal of bilayers, which leads to the stratum corneum becoming brittle. This can cause cracking within the stratum corneum. This leads to acid mantle damage and excessive TEWL. Flaking can result due to the lack of free water needed for the enzymes within the epidermis functioning well enough to break the desmosomes.

Cleansers for Aging Skin

The following types of cleansers are appropriate for aging skin:

- Neutral pH—correctly formulated for the skin type, not highly alkaline.
- Low surfactant, utilizing a nonionic surfactant, or biosurfactant. For example, a creamy cleanser or oil that converts to low foam. Refer to Table 7–1 on page 155 for a chart of nonionic surfactants and biosurfactants.
- Non-abrasive (no scrub ingredients).
- Easy to use.

Cleansers should be used twice a day for oilier skin types and at least nightly for drier skin types. A primary makeup remover should be used first for a complete cleanse. Use as a second cleanse in a professional esthetic treatment.

Exfoliants

Exfoliants are essential for use in professional treatments and are highly valuable in treating aging skin when used correctly at home. Caution must used with exfoliation, as overuse can occur quickly. Many clients think that an over-scrubbed skin is a clean skin, and this can cause more problems for the health of the skin. The two types of exfoliants are outlined in the sections that follow.

Physical or Mechanical: Scrubs:

Scrubs are manufactured particles or are taken from natural sources, for example, pumice, apricot seeds, and jojoba beads. Provide immediate results, can be irritating for compromised skin.

Chemical:

Proteolytic Enzymes: These enzymes digest proteins (proteolytic). To work, they need a catalyst, which is usually heat and water. They provide immediate results. The proteolytic enzymes include:

- Papain: derived from papaya
- Bromelain: derived from pineapple
- Cucurbita pepo ferment: derived from pumpkins

Acids: There are two types of acids: alpha hydroxy acids and beta hydroxy acids. All acids cause some damage to the stratum corneum because they set off a complex series of biochemical reactions in the skin. Some reactions can be positive, such as signaling the fibroblast to increase production of collagen. Other reactions can be undesirable, such as increasing the amount of melanin pigment within the skin. It is important for the esthetician to understand how to correctly analyze skin in order to avoid these harmful effects.

AHAs (Alpha Hydroxy Acids):   These acids are considered hydrophilic (attracted to water). The function of AHAs is to break desmosomes to facilitate faster cell turnover. AHAs are considered keratolytic due to this process. Commonly used AHAs include the following:

> There is up to an eight-day waiting period for desquamation of keratinocytes from an AHA peel, whereas enzymes provide a more immediate effect. Both are necessary for excellent results.

- **Glycolic acid:** derived from sugar cane, sugar beets, and synthetically manufactured, has a small molecular size (manufactured), low concentrations (2–5 percent) will facilitate a uniform exfoliation with no compromise of the skin's barrier; higher percentages are used in professional peels with variable pHs based on the manufacturer's formulation. Glycolic acid is also often used in *designer peels,* which are buffered multi-acid formulas specific to certain manufacturers. To facilitate better results, which include deeper penetration, be sure that the skin's barrier is always intact and healthy before using. This is why prepping the skin at least three weeks before a series of peels is so important. Good post-peel care is also important.[7]

- **Lactic acid:** derived from fermented sugar and synthetic sugar, the fermented sugar form is similar to NMF within the skin, suitable for compromised sensitive skin, is a mild tyrosinase inhibitor and pigment transfer inhibitor, and is often used as an humectant.
- **Mandelic acid:** used as an anti-bacterial agent as well as an exfoliant, effective for treatment of acne, has a larger molecular size which provides fewer negative side effects.

BHAs (Beta Hydroxy Acids): These acids are considered lipophilic (attracted to oil). The acids used in this category include the following:

- **Salicylic acid:** derived from willow bark, wintergreen leaves, and sweet birch, is anti-inflammatory, effective in lower percentages, useful for acne and rosacea, self-neutralizing, not for darker Fitzpatrick types, and is not known to stimulate fibroblasts.
- **Beta-lipohydroxy acid:** salicylic derivative which has slow diffusion, is less irritating, decreases bacteria, and is helpful for inflammatory acne.

pH:

Knowing the pH of the peel has been the guideline for effectiveness in the esthetic industry, but is not the only component of a peel that needs to be looked at. The type of acid or acids used as well as the buffering of the peel is as important as the pH. For example, you can have a multi-acid peel (also called a *designer peel)* with an acid content of 20 percent and a pH of 1.7 that is as gentle as a 30 percent lactic acid peel at a pH of 3.5 percent. This is possible through the delivery vehicle, buffering, and blend of acids used.

Chemical peeling is an important part of a healthy aging protocol, and it is important for an esthetician to understand the basic theory of use (Figures 7–1 and 7–2). There are three levels of peel depths: superficial, medium, and deep. See Chapter 6 for more details on professional chemical peeling.

Moisturizers and Multi-functional Formulations

The basic formulation of a moisturizer is an important part of maintaining and improving skin health. It is an often overlooked step, with estheticians going for the performance product first without initially getting the epidermis functioning optimally. In order for those performance ingredients to be effective, the epidermis must be well hydrated

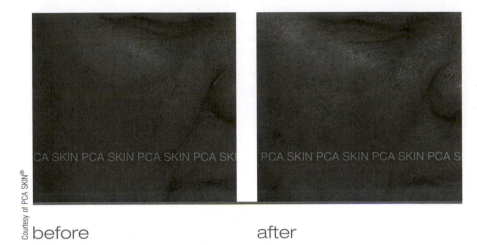

before   after

Figure 7–1 An example of a client's before and after using chemical exfoliation for treating hyperpigmentation and rough surface texture.

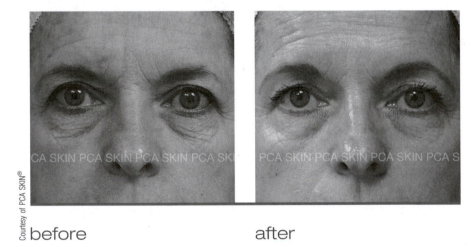

before   after

Figure 7–2 A client before and after using chemical exfoliation and daily home care for treating facial wrinkling, laxity, and dehydration.

with a minimal amount of TEWL. If there is damage to the lipid barrier, acid mantle, and enzymes are not functioning correctly, then subclinical inflammation may be present. Subclinical inflammation has been linked to many skin dysfunctions and skin aging.

A damaged stratum corneum can complete the repair process in 7–10 days based on the depth of the wound. Repair time is shortened when emollients are added to the skin. The best moisturizers are formulated to include ingredients that mimic the lipid and water content of the skin. These ingredients are called emollients and humectants. An emollient mimics the lipid bilayer, and a humectant mimics substances within the skin that are water soluble. Some common emollients and humectants are outlined in the sections that follow.

Hyaluronic Acid:

Holds 1,000 times its weight in water, and is an effective humectant. It is a major component, approximately 70 percent, of the GAGs found in the dermis that supply the fibroblast with nutrients, keeps skin plump and hydrated, functions as a delivery system, declines with age, and comes from natural or animal sources.

Essential Fatty Acids:

The building blocks of membranes, fats, and prostaglandins, known as omegas, biocompatible with cellular membranes and lipids, can treat disorders such as eczema, dermatitis, dry skin, and ichthyosis, and are extracted from plant and marine sources. Types of EFA used in skin care are:

- Linoleic acid
- Alpha-linoleic acid: kiwi seed oil, hemp oil, camelina oil
- Omega 3-6

The structure of NMF (natural moisture factor) is 40 percent amino acids, 30 percent cellular waste, 25 percent essential elements such as PCA, urea, sodium, calcium, potassium, magnesium, phosphate, chloride, lactate, and free amino acids.

Ceramides:

Make up 40 percent of the lipid bilayers, improve the permeability of the stratum corneum, repair the lipid barrier, improve hydration, slow TEWL, and help repair cell membranes. There are six types of ceramides within the skin. Common ceramides used in skin care are:

- Ceramide 3
- Ceraminol
- Omega-3 ceramide: from flax seed oil
- Omega-6 ceramide: from wheat germ, cottonseed, and evening primrose oil
- Vegetal ceramide: also an ingredient carrier
- Ceramide catiosphere: also a controlled release delivery system similar to a liposome.

Sphingolipids:

Biocompatible to the SC lipids, are a component of natural ceramides, sourced from wheat.

Free Fatty Acids:

Comprise 24 percent of the acid mantle, considered occlusive, slow TEWL, and maintain the pH of 5.5. There are two fatty acids important in skin care:

- Oleic acid: olive oil, acai, Brazilian palm berry, grape seed oil, sea buckthorn oil.
- Erucic acid: rapeseed oil, wallflower seed oil, mustard seed oil.

Silicones:

Used as thickeners, emollients, and lubricants, two types are used in skin care:

- Dimethicone: organic silicone, extracted from rocks and sand, used for barrier repair, slows TEWL, moisturizes skin, connects hyaluronic acid and mucopolysaccharides to skin proteins.[8]
- Cyclomethicone: acts as a wound healer, humectant, and connects hyaluronic acid to skin proteins.[9]

Algae:

Consists of nine amino acids, high bioavailability in the skin, type of algae determines the benefits such as antioxidant, wrinkle reduction, moisture, hydrator, emollient, and tissue renewal.

Sodium PCA:

Attracts water from the air, holds several times its weight in water, and imparts a temporary barrier as well as hydrating.

Calcium:

Regulates cell turnover, lipid formation, enhances barrier function, and helps to reduce cellular inflammation.

Amino Acids:

Forty percent of the NMF of the skin is composed of amino acids. These are the body's own natural humectants. Some common amino acids used in cosmetic formulations are:

- Glutamine
- Lysine
- Aspartic acid
- Threonine
- Arginine
- Proline

SUN PROTECTION

Sun protection is one of the most complicated and important aspects of skin care. UV radiation exposure is responsible for the extrinsic aging signs seen in skin. See Figure 7-3 for an example of the process. It is important to prevent the signs of aging, as well as protect against skin cancer. The directions that clients are given about sunscreen usage can be confusing, leading to misuse or non-use. This misinformation and the rise in skin cancer within the U.S. population have created a call for more education for the client. The esthetician is in the perfect position to provide that support.

In order to educate the client, it is important for the esthetician to understand some basic theory about SPF ratings, UV radiation exposure, and the damage it can do to the skin. The sections that follow outline the basics on ultraviolet radiation and how it affects the skin.

UVB (wavelengths of 290 nm):

Approximately 3.5 percent of the sun's rays reaching earth, considered more likely to cause skin cancer, DNA is considered a chromophore (target) of UV light. UVB is blocked by glass, and maximum strength of exposure happens between 10am and 3pm.[10] SPF stands for sun protection factor and only rates the amount of damage done by UVB radiation.

UVA1 (long wavelengths, 340–400nm) and UVA2 (short wavelengths, 320–340nm):

Make up 96 percent of the sun's rays reaching earth, which remain constant even with cloud cover, lead to immune system suppression within the skin, play a role in the development of melanomas, can penetrate glass, penetrate deeper into the skin causing damage to the dermis, responsible for photoaging signs including subclinical inflammation, increased MMPs, and pigmentation (Table 7–3).[11]

The universal standard quantity used to measure sunscreen effectiveness on application to the entire body is approximately 1 ounce or 30 mL. If the client is applying a powder such as mineral makeup, the amount would have to be 0.042 ounces or 1.2 grams, about the size of a 50-cent piece.

As of 2007 the FDA has proposed a new monograph for sunscreen labeling and testing. The rules as of 2010 have not been approved yet,

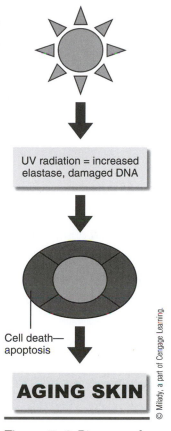

UV radiation = increased elastase, damaged DNA

Cell death— apoptosis

AGING SKIN

© Milady, a part of Cengage Learning.

Figure 7–3 Diagram of how UV damages the skin.

Table 7-3 Chart of UV wavelengths and penetration into the skin.

UV Wavelengths		Depth of Penetration into Skin
UVB 290 nm		Epidermis
UVA 320 nm	Penetrates glass	Dermis
Visible 400 nm		Hypodermis
Infrared 800 nm		Hypodermis

© Milady, a part of Cengage Learning.

The amount of sunscreen used on the face to meet the SPF rating needs to be about the size of a quarter, for the body the size of a shot glass. Do not forget that all exposed areas–neck, hands, and décolleté–all should have the size of a quarter applied. Studies have shown that clients only apply enough SPF to obtain about 1/3 of the protection stated on the label. This is another good reason to use a higher SPF.[12]

but manufacturers are asked to voluntarily comply. The new labeling rules are proposed as follows:

- Incorporate a new UVA protection rating system based on a 4-star system (Table 7–4). If a product has low UVA protection, the label would read *no UVA protection*.
- New testing would be implemented that measures the sunscreen's ability to block UVA and prevent the skin from developing persistent pigment darkening (PPD).
- Add a *warnings statement* in the drug facts box which states *UV exposure from the sun increases the risk of skin cancer, premature skin aging, and other skin damage. It is important to decrease UV exposure by limiting time in the sun, wearing protective clothing, and using sunscreen.*
- SPF labels would be able to read SPF 50+ instead of the recognized SPF 30+. The legitimate range would then be SPF 2 to SPF 50+.
- Terminology such as *sunblock, waterproof, chemical free, natural, all-day protection, extended wear,* and *non-chemical* are no longer

Table 7-4 Proposed UVA protection rating system based on a 4 star system.

	Proposed sunscreen rating system
☆	1 star- low UVA protection
☆☆	2 stars- medium UVA protection
☆☆☆	3 stars- high UVA protection
☆☆☆☆	4 stars-highest available UVA protection

© Milady, a part of Cengage Learning.

allowed. New terms allowed are *water resistant* and *very water resistant*.

- Allows new combinations of active ingredients.

This has been an ongoing and hotly debated process within the FDA, and manufacturers may not have to comply for up to two years after passing. This puts the responsibility on the client to understand the currently approved sunscreen ingredients to make a safe informed decision.

Chemical Sunscreens

Chemical sunscreens absorb the UV radiation and traditionally only protected against UVB. These ingredients can result in further ROS (reactive oxygen species free radicals) being created or reactions within the sunscreen that deactivate other chemicals. Usually the absorbed UVR is released as heat at a longer wavelength with no damage.[13] Recently, new formulations of chemical sunscreens that also absorb UVA have been available. Common sunscreen ingredients are described in the sections that follow.

Chemical UVB-Absorbing Sunscreens

Para-aminobenzoic Acid: Highly sensitizing; most professional-level sunscreens do not contain this ingredient. Names used are:[15,16]

- PABA
- Padimate O, which is the same as Octyl Dimethyl PABA
- Aminobenzoic acid
- Amyl dimethyl PABA
- Glyceryl aminobenzoate
- Glyceryl PABA
- Ethyl-4-bis aminobenzoate
- Ethyl dihydroxypropyl PABA

Chemical sunscreens can be unstable. For example, studies have shown that avobenzone has a decrease in effectiveness of 36 percent when exposed to 15 minutes of UVR.[14] A good formulation will always have additional antioxidants and other sunscreen ingredients to be effective.

Cinnamates: The most commonly used sunscreen ingredients, UVB maximum absorption of 310 nm, poorly soluble in water, often included in water-resistant formulations, can cause allergic reactions. Names used are:

- 2-methoxy ethyl-p-methoxycinnamate
- Octyl methoxycinnamate (OMC)
- Diethanolamine-p-methoxycinnamate

Salicylates: Maximum UVB absorption of 310 nm, stable, non-sensitizing, water insoluble, and used in multiple ingredient formulations. Names used are:

- Octyl salicylate
- Homosalate
- Triethanolamine salicylate
- Phenylbenzimidazole sulfonic acid

Chemical UVA-Absorbing Sunscreens

Benzophenones:

Maximum absorption range is 320 nm to 350 nm, best blocker of short-wave UVA2, used in approximately 30 percent of sunscreens on market, can cause photoallergic contact dermatitis, systemic absorption can happen when applied in large amounts, not recommended for children.[17] Names used are:

- Avobenzone
- Dioxybenzone
- Sulisobenzone
- Tetrahydroxybenzophenone
- Benzophenone-6
- Oxybenzone
- Benzophenone-1
- Benzophenone-12

Methyl Anthranilate:

Absorption maximum at 340 nm, less effective than benzophenones, not widely used.

Parsol 1789:

Absorption maximum at 355 nm, approved by FDA in 1990s, can cause photoallergic contact dermatitis, old formulation was unstable, new stable forms became available in 2007 as Helioplex (Neutrogena) and Active Photobarrier Complex (Aveeno). Names used:

- Butyl methoxydibenzoylmethane
- Benzophenone-3

Mexoryl SX:

Not as effective as formula used in Europe Mexoryl XL, water soluble, suitable for everyday use, organic filter effective on shorter UVA, more stable than avobenzone.

Physical Sunscreens

Physical sunscreens scatter and reflect UV radiation rather than absorb it. They are considered to be broad spectrum protection, which means protection from UVB, UVA, visible light, and infrared radiation. Physical sunscreens are recommended for high-intensity exposure such as the beach or high altitudes and are safe for sensitive skin.

One concern of these physical sunscreens is the free radical damage that can be done within the skin if the ingredient (titanium dioxide) is poorly formulated and penetrates into the skin. Zinc oxide is more stable and a good formulation will coat the physical blocks with dimethicone or silicone for stability. Nanoparticle size concerns have been voiced by many in the scientific field due to the hypothesis of penetration into the stratum corneum. This nanotechnology has been in use for over 20 years and is considered safe. The answer that addresses many concerns is that, although the zinc has been micronized, it is still too large to penetrate the skin due to the other aspects of the formulation.

Titanium Dioxide (Ti02):

Reflects UVA and UVB, non-irritating, can cause free radical damage in skin if absorbed.

Zinc Oxide (Zn0):

Blocks more UVA and UVB radiation, stable, non-irritating, comes in nanoparticle formulations. Is frequently used in formulations with chemical sunscreens.

▪ PERFORMANCE INGREDIENTS

Antioxidants

> The FDA specifically regulates the combinations of sunscreen ingredients due to the reactivity of many formulas.

Antioxidants are a necessity for treating aging skin. The range of antioxidants can include water-soluble and oil-soluble vitamins, essential oils, plant polyphenols, flavinoids, bioflavonoids, and radical scavengers manufactured in a lab.

Antioxidants act as free radical scavengers and help prevent cell damage before it happens. Traditional antioxidants act upon the free radicals (ROS) by chemically converting them to water. Chapter 4 contains additional information on the free radical theory of aging and the importance of antioxidants.

Spin Traps

Spin traps are considered nitrones and are *smart* antioxidants. They effectively slow down and trap the free radicals before they can do any damage.

Ingredient names to look for in formulas are:[18]

- n-tert-butyl-alpha-phenylnitrone
- 3,5-dibromo-4-nitrosobenzenesulfonic acid
- 2-methyl-2-nitrosopropane
- Alpha-n-t-butylnitrone
- 2,4,6-tri-t-butylnitrosobenzone
- 2,2,6,6-tetramethylpiperidine-n-oxyl (tempo)
- 5,5-dimethyl-1-pyrroline n-oxide
- Nitrosodisulfonic acid
- 3,3,5,5-tetramethylpyrroline n-oxide

Vitamin E

Vitamin E is known as an oil-soluble antioxidant and has two groups, tocopherols and tocotrienols. Vitamin E needs water-soluble vitamins such as C to be an effective antioxidant and is usually combined with other ingredients in a formulation.

Tocopherols are considered esters and are used in such formulations as:[19]

- Tocopheryl acetate
- d-tocopheryl glucoside: emollient, vit e with glycerin
- Tocopheryl linoleate: emollient and humectant
- Tocopheryl phosphate: delivery system
- Sodium tocopheryl phosphate: new water-soluble formulation
- Tocotrienols are less widely used, but new research has showed that this form of vitamin E may have more potent antioxidant benefits and have better skin absorption. Tocotrienol is found in palm oil, rice bran oil, oat, barley, and rye.

Vitamin C:

Is a water-soluble antioxidant, important for collagen stimulation, wound healing, nutrient absorption, and melanin suppression. Vitamin C is oxidized quickly and is active only for a short time. The body does not make vitamin C; it must be supplied through diet, supplementation, and topical application. There are several types used in skin care formulations; ascorbic acid is considered the natural form of vitamin C, has a short shelf life and is chirally correct. Vitamin C can be irritating due to the acidic pH.

Ascorbyl Tetraisopalmitate: Lipid soluble and stable, less acidic and irritating, easily passes through lipid bilayers to reach cells. Ascorbyl tetraisopalmitate has a good shelf life.

Ascorbyl Palmitate (ester): Lipid-soluble form widely used, combined with palmitic acid, acts as an antioxidant, combined with amino acids and L-ascorbic acid to strengthen connective tissue and vascular walls.

Magnesium Ascorbyl Phosphate: Water soluble, low irritation, stable, improves collagen synthesis, effective in lower concentrations by causing the cells to uptake a higher dose due to the magnesium; expensive ingredient used in professional skin care.

Ubiquinone–Coenzyme Q10:

Oil-soluble antioxidant found in mitochondria of cells, helps generate ATP, helps reduce MMPs. Synthetic form is ubiquinone, also known as idebenone, which is water soluble.

Ergothioneine:

Amino acid derived from mushrooms or animal tissues, more effective than idebenone in stopping lipid peroxidation, keratinocytes have receptors that allow ergothioneine to penetrate into cell.

Green Tea:

High level of polyphenols, inhibits MMP enzymes, reduces small capillary clumping, inflammation, and erythema, and has photoprotective properties.

Alpha Lipoic Acid:

Known as thioctic acid, both oil and water soluble, can fight free radicals both inside and outside the cell, necessary for glucose to convert to ATP, works with other antioxidants by converting the vitamins back to an active state after the free radical has been stopped.

Lutein:

Has the ability to protect the skin from UV by absorbing blue light; some of the sources are nasturtium, Indian cress, and monk cress.

Superoxide dismutase (SOD):

An enzyme found in the body that acts as a free radical scavenger, prevents lipid peroxidation, and helps the body use zinc, copper, and manganese.[20]

Peptides

Synthetic peptides are exciting new ingredients that have different effects on the skin based on the type of peptide used. Peptides are the links between amino acids and regulate or influence cell activity. Proteins consist of approximately 50–plus amino acids linked in a chain and then arranged in a globular form. This is considered a polypeptide.[21] The length and composition of the peptide chain determines the activity.

Common classifications of peptides include:[22]

- Polypeptide: single chain of amino acids
- Tripeptides: chain of three amino acids
- Tetrapeptides: chain of four amino acids
- Pentapeptides: chain of five amino acids
- Oligopeptides: chains of 2–20 amino acids
- Lipopeptides: attached to proteins and lipids

The peptides that are used in skin care formulations are synthetic peptides in various combinations. The goal of these peptides is to communicate with cells and direct them to act in a certain way. Some commonly used peptides are:

- Collagen synthesis stimulators: Matrixyl (palmitoyl pentapeptide-3), Matrixyl 3000 (palmitoyl oligopeptide), tetrapeptide-3 and 7 (Rigin)
- GAG and elastin synthesis: copper peptides (GHK)
- Wrinkle smoothing: Acetyl hexapeptide-3 (Argireline)
- Pigment inhibiting: Melanostat, Lumixyl, sea beet peptide, sea fennel
- Antioxidant: Glutathione

Anti-Pigmentation Agents

Pigmentation problems are always challenging. Treating this condition requires ingredients that work at multiple steps in the process of creating melanin. It can take up to 28 weeks to see an improvement in pigment with client protocol use mandatory. Besides the active ingredients listed in the sections that follow, sunscreen is important as well as antioxidant protection. See Chapter 5 for an explanation on how melanin is formed. The two categories of ingredients that are needed to treat pigmentation disorders are tyrosinase inhibitors and melanosome transfer inhibitors.

Tyrosinase Inhibitors
Interrupt the enyzematic action that causes pigmentation to form with in the melanocyte.

Magnesium Ascorbyl Phosphate: See description of vitamin C.

Arbutin: Effective at low concentrations, extracted from the bearberry plant, also used as an antioxidant.

Azelaic acid: Better suited for Fitzpatrick types 4–6, low irritation, works on abnormal melanocytes and post-inflammatory pigmentation. Also used as an acne treatment by inhibiting 5a-reductase.[23]

Glucosamine: Interferes with the formation of tyrosinase, works well with niacinamide.

Paper mulberry: Studies show that in the correct concentration it is as effective as hydroquinone and kojic acid. Effective at lower concentrations than the usual concentration hydroquinone and kojic acid. Comes from plant source.[24]

Glabridin: Main component of licorice extract, anti-inflammatory, antioxidant, and inhibits tyrosinase; also used as a melanin inhibitor.

Aloesin: Sourced from aloe vera, has been demonstrated to be have a stronger inhibitory effect on tyrosinase than arbutin and kojic acid.

Kojic Acid: Derived from fungus, it is used in food, suppresses tyrosinase, is stable, more effective when combined with glycolic acid, and has a high sensitizing potential at 2.5 percent level.

Hydroquinone: Used in concentrations of 2 percent OTC and 4 percent by prescription, known to be toxic to cells and has potential to discolor the skin, it is banned in Europe and Asia. It is a tyrosinase inhibitor and cytotoxic to melanocytes.[25]

Melanosome Transfer Inhibitors
Interupt the transfer of pigment granules to keratinocytes.

Niacinamide: Vitamin B3, anti-inflammatory, antioxidant, inhibits transfer of melanosomes to keratinocytes up to 68 percent. Used in popular OTC cosmetic lines and as a treatment for acne. A 4 percent concentration has been shown to have equal results as 1 percent clindamycin.[26]

Soy: Soymilk-derived protein (STI and BBI) reverses skin pigmentation and prevents further melanosome transfer; pasteurized soymilk ingredients are ineffective.

Anti-inflammatory Agents

Inflammation has been shown to be the basis of many skin conditions and disorders, with a large role in aging skin, including rosacea. Controlled wounding induces an inflammation response that is a benefit to skin, but long-term uncontrolled inflammation needs to be reduced. Some ingredients used topically that can help are outlined in the sections that follow.

German Chamomile:

Suppresses inflammation and leukocyte infiltration, improves texture and elasticity, and has mild antioxidant properties.

Aloe Vera:

Used in treatment for burns and wounds, components of aloe such as salicylates, magnesium lactate, polysaccharides, and C-glycosyl have anti-inflammatory properties.

Cucumber Extract:

Emollient, soothing, contains high amounts of amino acids which help the acid mantle. Shikimate dehydrogenase, an enzyme extracted from the pulp, has anti-inflammatory properties.[27]

Licorice Extract:

Glycyrrhizin is the active component with anti-inflammatory activity, has been used to treat contact dermatitis, pruritus, seborrheic dermatitis, and psoriasis, due to its cortisone-like effects.

Selenium:

An essential element found in spa mineral water, helps the body form glutathione, and prevents the production of inflammatory cytokines leading to decreased inflammation; topical absorption is only possible with L-selenomethionine.

Colloidal Oatmeal:

Compound made from dehulled oats ground into fine powder, effective in the management of pediatric atopic dermatitis and is recognized by the FDA as an effective skin protector, it can decrease transepidermal water loss (TEWL), has antioxidant activity, hydrates the skin, and provides a protective barrier. Contains a new group of polyphenols called avenanthramides, which are the strongest antioxidants found in nature and show potent anti-inflammatory activity.[28]

Pycnogenol:

Extracted from the maritime pine tree, known as a bioflavonoid that helps protect vitamin C within the body, reduces inflammation, slowing new growth of capillaries from existing capillaries (angiogenesis). Good for vascular conditions.

Grape Seed Extract:

Known as a bioflavonoid, reduces inflammation and blood platelet clumping, reduces oxidative stress, and is an oleic acid, which helps prevent TEWL.

Anti-aging Ingredients

Ingredient manufacturers are continually releasing new and interesting ingredients created for the anti-aging market. Some may have profound effects on the skin. Many ingredients are untested and long-term efficacy is not always proven. There are proven essential ingredients needed to stimulate the fibroblasts to make collagen, elastin, and glycosaminoglycans. These ingredients are vitally important for treating aging skin. They are:

- Vitamin C
- Growth factors
- Iron
- Silicon, magnesium, calcium
- Essential fatty acids
- Bioflavonoids
- Zinc
- Amino acids (proline and lysine)
- Vitamin A
- Copper peptides

Growth Factor:

Epidermal growth factor (EGF) acts as a chemical messenger between cells that regulate cell growth, proliferation and differentiation, the synthetic ingredient is created from bovine sources, cultured epidermal cells, placental cells, human foreskin, colostrums and some plants, it is required for collagen repair, replacement, production and distribution, wound healing, cell, blood vessel growth. Insulin-like growth factor (IGF) is polypeptides and plays a role in cell proliferation and inhibition of cell death; it is expensive, at about $30,000 per gram. Transforming growth factors-beta (TGF-β1, TGF-β2, TGF-β3) are multi-function peptides that control cell differentiation, cell proliferation, and cellular transformation.[29]

Retinoids:

Compounds derived from vitamin A that include retinol, tretinoin, tazarotene, adapalene, and retinaldehyde and beta carotene. Skin cells have retinoic acid receptors which then change the vitamin A compound to retinol, then retinaldehyde, then to retinoic acid, which is metabolized by the mitochondria. Retinoids reduce oxidative stress, activate vitamin A receptor in cells, restore cellular balance, increase cell growth and differentation, inhibit MMPs, and prevent the loss of collagen from UV exposure. Retinaldehyde has been shown to repair collagen and elastin damage from UVA exposure in concentrations of 0.05 percent.[30] Retinoids are essential anti-aging ingredients.

Beta Glucan:

Reduces wrinkle size and depth via fibroblast stimulation and collagen deposition, penetrates into the dermis well, sourced from oats.

Malus Dosmestica:

New anti-aging ingredient that protects stem cells from UV, promotes longer stem cell lifespan, and reduces the appearance of wrinkles.

Phycojuvenine:

Stimulates keratinocyte and fibroblast stem cells, reduces wrinkle depth, and shortens wound healing time.

Mexican bamboo:

Increases sirtuin activity (anti-aging enzymes that protect cells); anti-inflammatory and antioxidant.

Ingredients That Cause Concern

There is much misinformation about safe cosmetic ingredients; even estheticians are confused. Listed in the sections that follow are some of the most common ingredients that clients are concerned about.

Case Study

Let's continue our case study and include a home care regimen.

Client: 42-year-old female

Skin type: Combination-Fitzpatrick Type 2

Conditions: Photodamage (hyperpigmentation), fine lines (stage 1 aging), dehydration, hyperkeratinized (dead skin cell buildup), comedones (blackheads)

Assessment: Client has identified with wrong skin type thus using the wrong home care products, high stress levels are impacting hydration and texture issues in the skin. Perimenopausal symptoms are adding to skin condition. Fitzpatrick type is good for most clinical treatments.

Goal for home care: Increase desquamation to reduce fine lines, increase fibroblast stimulation, hydration (free water in the epidermis), suppress melanin production (inhibit tyrosinase production, reduce melanosome transfer), reduce inflammation, increase free radical protection.

Home care regimen:

AM: Hydration and Protection

Cleanse: Gentle low surfactant cleanser

Tone: Tonic with peptides or antioxidants

Serum: Antioxidant serum, possible ingredients:

Magnesium Ascorbyl Phosphate—Vitamin C

Spin Traps

PhytoCellTec

Soy

Moisturize/Protect: balanced humectant/emollient cream for combination skin with possible ingredients:

Free fatty acids such as acai oil

Essential fatty acids such as flax seed oil

Pycnogenol

Algae

Soy

Protection should be at least an SPF 30, physical sunscreen—zinc oxide

PM: Correct and Repair

Cleanse: Low surfactant cleanser for combination skin

Tone: Tonic with peptides or antioxidants

Serum: Tyrosinase and melanosome transfer inhibitor

Magnesium Ascorbyl Phosphate—Vitamin C

Kojic acid

Alpha arbutin

Treatment Cream: balanced humectants/emollient for combination skin with at least .25 percent of retinol or .5 percent of retinaldehyde, essential fatty acids, free fatty acids, antioxidants, soy and possible growth factors.

This program should be reevaluated within three months as professional treatments progress. If the client is moving into a series of peels, a prepping product with AHAs in it should be used for at least two weeks (Fitzpatrick 1–3), or four to eight weeks (Fitzpatrick 4–6).

Parabens

Parabens are used as preservatives and are derived from the processing of petroleum. They are anti-fungal and anti-bacterial. They are found in foods such as cheeses, beverages, processed meats, and pickled foods. They are also found naturally in blueberries and grape seed.

There are four different types of parabens:

- Methylparaben: anti-fungal
- Propylparaben: anti-fungal, used in foods
- Butylparaben
- Ethylparaben

To be effective, parabens are usually used at low concentrations (usually .01 to .03 percent) and were reviewed for safety in 2005 by the Cosmetic Ingredient Review board.

Health Concerns   Health concerns were raised in 2004 with the publication of a study that detected parabens in breast tumors. The study did not show that parabens cause cancer, and it did not study paraben levels in normal tissue. The questions were brought up about the endocrine disruption possibly caused by parabens due to their ability to mimic estrogen within the body. High levels of endocrine disruptors do have health risks; it is not known at this time if parabens accumulate within the body.

Phthalates and Bisphenol A (BPA)

Phthalates are a group of chemicals used to soften plastics, and BPA is a chemical used to make plastics stronger. Both are used in food and cosmetic packaging. There is much concern over the use of this group of chemicals due to health concerns that can result in endocrine disruption, including thyroid function. Phthalates and BPA can be used in a wide variety of products such as:

- Enteric coatings of pharmaceuticals
- Fragrances
- Nutritional supplements
- Building materials
- Glue and adhesives
- Food containers
- Floor tiles
- Cosmetics
- Liquid hand soap
- Plastic bottles
- Baby toys
- Baby bottles

Health Concerns   There are significant health concerns with phthalates and BPA that are only recently being studied. Americans are commonly exposed to this chemical in their environment as well as directly from diet. Phthalates easily evaporate and leach into the environment and into food. Fatty foods such as milk, butter, and meats are a source. Children are especially vulnerable to exposure, and body care products with phthalates are a source of exposure.[31] BPA is found in the lining of food containers, plastic baby bottles, and PVC. Contamination can happen with the breakdown of plastics within the environment. The method of direct human contamination has not been proven at this time, but studies have shown BPA in the urine of human subjects.

Health concerns focus on endocrine disruption, which can impact insulin resistance and obesity as well as sexual development in children. Also of concern is the impact on the liver, asthma, and allergies.

> Plastic water bottles contain PETE, which is not a phthalate. It is easily recycled. There is some concern about endocrine disruption through leaching of phthalates, which is primarily dependent on the method and duration of storage.

> > > Top Ten Tips to Take to the Clinic

1. Harsh surfactants in cleansers can disrupt the acid mantle.
2. Absorption of ingredients in the skin must be facilitated by delivery systems such as liposomes, nanosomes, low molecular weight, and other treatment applications.
3. Essential products are important when trying to improve skin.
4. Performance ingredients are used when trying to correct aging skin conditions.
5. Sun protection is mandatory when treating aging skin.
6. UV radiation accounts for 80 percent of signs of aging.
7. Ingredients that cause concern are parabens, phthalates, and BPA.
8. Ingredients that cause concern are thought to be endocrine disruptors.
9. It is the frequency and dosage of active ingredients that can affect the skin.
10. Some form of preservative should always be used in products.

Chapter Review Questions

1. What is the FDA definition of cosmetics?
2. How far does UVA penetrate skin?
3. Does SPF rating indicate protection against all UV radiation?

4. What is the difference between a chemical and physical sunscreen ingredient?

5. Have parabens been proven to be toxic?

References

1. Barrett-Hill, F. (2010). *Cosmetic Chemistry*. Whangaparaoa, New Zealand: Virtual Beauty Corporation Ltd.
2. Barrett-Hill, F. (2010). *Cosmetic Chemistry*. Whangaparaoa, New Zealand: Virtual Beauty Corporation Ltd.
3. Barrett-Hill, F. (2010). *Cosmetic Chemistry*. Whangaparaoa, New Zealand: Virtual Beauty Corporation Ltd.
4. Barrett-Hill, F. (2010). *Cosmetic Chemistry*. Whangaparaoa, New Zealand: Virtual Beauty Corporation Ltd.
5. Barrett-Hill, F. (2010). *Cosmetic Chemistry*. Whangaparaoa, New Zealand: Virtual Beauty Corporation Ltd.
6. Baumann, L. MD., Saghari, S. MD., Weisburg, E. MS. (2009). *Cosmetic Dermatology: Principles and Practice*, 2nd Edition. New York: McGraw Hill Medical.
7. Barrett-Hill, F. (2010). *Cosmetic Chemistry*. Whangaparaoa, New Zealand: Virtual Beauty Corporation Ltd.
8. Pillai, R., et al. Anti-Wrinkle Therapy: Significant New Findings in the Non-Invasive Cosmetic Treatment of Skin Wrinkles with Beta-Glucan.
9. Pillai, R., et al. Anti-Wrinkle Therapy: Significant New Findings in the Non-Invasive Cosmetic Treatment of Skin Wrinkles with Beta-Glucan.
10. Marks, R. (August 2004). *"The Stratum Corneum Barrier: The Final Frontier."* Journal of Neurology, Vol. 134:2017S–2021S.
11. Marks, R. (August 2004). *"The Stratum Corneum Barrier: The Final Frontier."* Journal of Neurology, Vol. 134:2017S–2021S.
12. Marks, R. (August 2004). *"The Stratum Corneum Barrier: The Final Frontier."* Journal of Neurology, Vol. 134:2017S–2021S.
13. Marks, R. (August 2004). *"The Stratum Corneum Barrier: The Final Frontier."* Journal of Neurology, Vol. 134:2017S–2021S.
14. Marks, R. (August 2004). *"The Stratum Corneum Barrier: The Final Frontier."* Journal of Neurology, Vol. 134:2017S–2021S.
15. Barrett-Hill, F. (2010). *Cosmetic Chemistry*. Whangaparaoa, New Zealand: Virtual Beauty Corporation Ltd.
16. Baumann, L. MD., Saghari, S. MD., Weisburg, E. MS. (2009). *Cosmetic Dermatology: Principles and Practice*, 2nd Edition. New York: McGraw Hill Medical.

17. Baumann, L. MD., Saghari, S. MD., Weisburg, E. (2009). *Cosmetic Dermatology: Principles and Practice*, 2nd Edition. New York: McGraw Hill Medical.
18. Barrett-Hill, F. (2010). *Cosmetic Chemistry*. Whangaparaoa, New Zealand: Virtual Beauty Corporation Ltd.
19. Barrett-Hill, F. (2010). *Cosmetic Chemistry*. Whangaparaoa, New Zealand: Virtual Beauty Corporation Ltd.
20. Barrett-Hill, F. (2010). *Cosmetic Chemistry*. Whangaparaoa, New Zealand: Virtual Beauty Corporation Ltd.
21. Barrett-Hill, F. (2010). *Cosmetic Chemistry*. Whangaparaoa, New Zealand: Virtual Beauty Corporation Ltd.
22. Barrett-Hill, F. (2010). *Cosmetic Chemistry*. Whangaparaoa, New Zealand: Virtual Beauty Corporation Ltd.
23. Barrett-Hill, F. (2010). *Cosmetic Chemistry*. Whangaparaoa, New Zealand: Virtual Beauty Corporation Ltd.
24. Barrett-Hill, F. (2010). *Cosmetic Chemistry*. Whangaparaoa, New Zealand: Virtual Beauty Corporation Ltd.
25. Barrett-Hill, F. (2010). *Cosmetic Chemistry*. Whangaparaoa, New Zealand: Virtual Beauty Corporation Ltd.
26. Barrett-Hill, F. (2010). *Cosmetic Chemistry*. Whangaparaoa, New Zealand: Virtual Beauty Corporation Ltd.
27. Root, L. (2009). *The Skin Care Professional's Chemistry and Ingredient Handbook*. Esthetic Education Resource LLC.
28. Root, L. (2009). *The Skin Care Professional's Chemistry and Ingredient Handbook*. Esthetic Education Resource LLC.
29. Root, L. (2009). *The Skin Care Professional's Chemistry and Ingredient Handbook*. Esthetic Education Resource LLC.
30. Boisnic, S., Branchet-Gumila, M., Le Charpentier, Y., Segard, C. (1999). "Repair of UVA-induced Elastic Fiber and Collagen Damage by .05% Retinaldehyde cream in an ex vivo Human Skin Model," *Dermatology* (suppl 1): 43–48.
31. Sathyanarayana, S., Karr, C. J., Lozano, P., *et al*. (February 2008). "Baby care products: possible sources of infant phthalate exposure". Pediatrics 121 (2): e260–8.

Bibliography

Barrett-Hill, F. (2004). *Advanced Skin Analysis*, 2nd Edition. Whangaparaoa, New Zealand: Virtual Beauty Corporation Ltd.

Boisnic, S., Branchet-Gumila, M., Le Charpentier, Y., Segard, C. (1999). "Repair of UVA-induced Elastic Fiber and Collagen

Damage by .05% Retinaldehyde Cream in an Ex vivo Human Skin Model, *Dermatology* (suppl 1): 43–48.

Calafat, A. M., Kuklenyik Z., Reidy J. A., Caudill S. P., Ekong J., Needham L. L. (2005). "Urinary Concentrations of Bisphenol A and 4-nonylphenol in a Human Reference Population," *Environmental Health Perspectives* 113 (4): 391–5.

Kashiwagi, K., Furuno, N., Kitamura, S., Ohta, S., Sugihara, K., Utsumi, K., Hanada, H., Taniguchi, K., et al. (2009). "Disruption of Thyroid Hormone Function by Environmental Pollutants," *Journal of Health Science* 55: 147.

Michalun, N., Michalun, M. V. (2010). *Milady's Skin Care and Cosmetic Ingredients Dictionary*, 3rd Edition. Clifton Park, NY: Cengage Learning.

Pugliese, P. MD. (2001). *Physiology of the Skin II*. Carol Stream, IL: Allured Publishing.

Websites

http://www.fda.gov

    Look for SEC.201 [21.U.S.C. 321] - Federal Food Drug and Cosmetic Act

www.sederma.fr/Actives/Matrixyl.htm

www.cosmeticsbusiness.com

Nutrition, Supplements, & Fitness

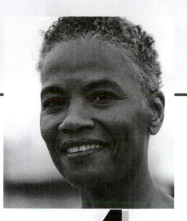

SECTION CONTENTS

Section **4**

Aesthetic Medical Treatment Options

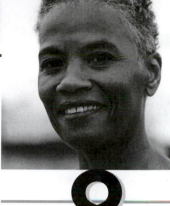

Chapter 8

Key Terms

American National
    Standards
    Institute (ANSI)
anaphylactic
fractionated laser

ground state
laser
nonsteroidal anti-
    inflammatory
    drug (NSAID)

pigmented lesions
vascular lesions

Learning Objectives

After completing this chapter, you will be able to:

1. Explain how lasers work.

2. Describe the aesthetic medicinal treatment options available for your client.

3. Explain the esthetician's role in aesthetic medicine.

INTRODUCTION

The role of an esthetician in an aesthetic medical practice is challenging and exciting. Having access to the latest technology and treatments can be fulfilling. It can also be hard to integrate the holistic esthetic model that is the core of the esthetic profession into a medical practice. As this industry continues to grow, the role of the esthetician is becoming more and more important.

Some treatment options can be performed by an esthetician under a physician's direction and others cannot. It is important for the esthetician to understand the treatments available, both invasive and non-invasive, in order to work in the medical environment as well as advise clients who come in for comprehensive healthy aging programs.

Always check with your state licensing board to determine your scope of practice. Even if you work for a doctor, you are responsible for working within the licensing scope, and you can be liable for anything outside that scope even with supervision.

OPTIONS FOR NON-INVASIVE TREATMENT

Non-invasive treatments are treatments that do not require a long recovery period. Non-invasive techniques may require multiple treatments to see results, and the treatments may have side effects. These treatments are not without some pain, but technology and client care protocols are getting better.

LASERS AND IPL

Lasers and intense pulsed light (IPL) technology offer some of the most exciting and effective treatments for skin that have ever been used. Lasers have been used in medical treatments since the early 1960s.

Laser surgery is definitely in the medical realm and outside the esthetician's scope of practice unless supervised by a physician. The exciting part of laser technology is that it is getting safer and less invasive. Currently some states allow IPL technology for use in non–doctor-supervised clinics, but this is controversial and is being reviewed by many regulating boards.

Understanding Lasers

laser
acronym for *light amplification by the stimulated emission of radiation;* laser technology emits photons in a coherent beam. A laser has three parts: *energy source, active medium,* and *optical cavity.*

The word **laser** is actually an acronym that stands for *light amplification by the stimulated emission of radiation.* This technology is based on the theories of Max Planck and Albert Einstein. Planck's theory states that the nucleus of an atom is positively charged and that the orbit is negatively charged. The closer the electron is to the nucleus of an atom, the lower the energy. This is called the **ground state**. When energy is introduced to the atom, it will cause negatively charged electrons to jump farther from the nucleus and create an excited state. The electron wants to return to the ground state, so it must give off the extra energy in the form of photons.

Einstein's theory expands on Planck's and states that when the photons created crash into an excited system, they create multiple photons of the same wavelength, building a large amount of light energy in one wavelength. The wavelength is determined by the substance that these photons reflect from. For example, the mineral alexandrite will create wavelengths of 755 nm.

ground state
state of lease possible energy or zero energy point.

How Lasers Work

Laser technology emits photons in a coherent beam. A laser has three parts: *energy source, active medium,* and *optical cavity.*

Energy Source: This is the energy that excites the active medium; usually this is electricity.

Active Medium: This is a solid, gas, or liquid that is excited by the energy source, releasing photons that determine wavelength.

Optical Cavity: This is also called a *resonator,* an area equipped with a high-reflectance mirror and a partial-reflectance mirror. A photon cascade bounces off the mirrors and gains strength until it pushes through the partial-reflectance mirror.

Laser light is monochromatic and is emitted in a narrow beam, created by energizing the lasing medium (for example, ruby, alexandrite, or CO_2) in the laser's optical cavity and then bouncing the beam off two mirrors. One mirror is fully reflective; the other is partially reflective. This allows the partially reflective mirror to shutter open and closed to release the photons, thus producing a laser beam. *Q-switching* is a method of providing intense laser pulses by utilizing a mechanical or electrical q-switch. How this energy is produced and applied to the skin makes a difference in the type of results you will get. Figure 8–1 illustrates the components of a laser.

Lasers' Effect on Skin

Different lasers target different components in the skin. This is accomplished by a process called selective photothermolysis, in which laser wavelengths heat the skin and are absorbed by the target chromophore, which is the part of the molecule that absorbs or detects light energy. For example, oxyhemoglobin (blood), melanin, or water have a specific chromophore which will attract a certain wavelength (Figure 8–2).

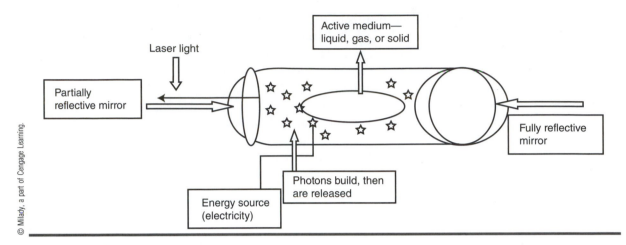

Figure 8–1 Components of a laser.

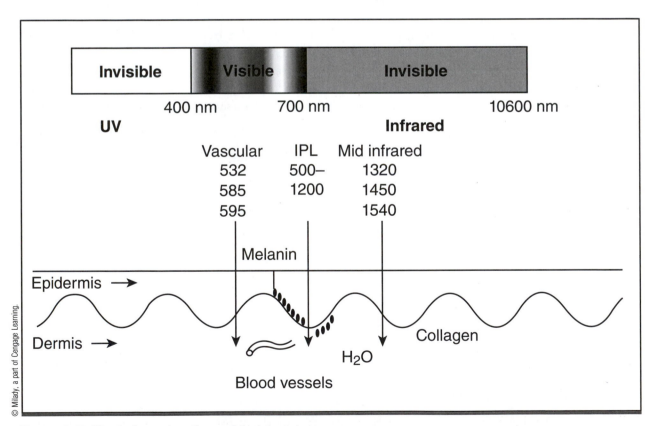

Figure 8–2 Chart of wavelengths and their targets.

Skin Type	UV Exposure	Characteristics	Possible Reactions
Skin Type I	Always burns, never tans; usually burns within 10–15 minutes	White, very fair, red or blond hair, blue eyes, freckles likely	Sensitivity to topical products, the environment, heat, cold, and wind
Skin Type II	Burns easily, tans minimally; usually burns within 30–40 minutes	Fair-skinned, blue, green, or hazel eyes, blond, dishwater blond, or red hair	Rarely develop post-inflammatory pigmentation, least defense against UV damage
Skin Type III	Sometimes burns, gradually tans; usually burns within 60–70 minutes	Cream-white, fair with any eye or hair color, very common coloring	
Skin Type IV	Rarely burns, gradually tans	Brown skin, brown eyes, Mediterranean, southern European, Hispanic	More susceptible to pigmentation problems and keloid scarring, greater defense against environmental and UV damage
Skin Type V	Tans	Dark brown skin, brown-black hair, brown eyes, Asian, Indian, some Africans	
Skin Type VI	Tans well	Black skin, black hair, brown-black eyes, Africans	

Figure 8–3 Fitzpatrick skin types and possible reactions.

When lasers generate enough heat, they can vaporize or destroy tissues. Pulses of power measured in milliseconds help protect the surrounding tissue. This allows for a controlled cool-down period. There is no single type of laser that will produce results for all skin conditions (Figure 8–3). Lasers are classified by the medium used to produce the specific wavelengths. These classes are *solid state, semiconductor, gas,* and *dye.*

LASER SAFETY

Estheticians must be fully trained in laser safety; ignorance is not acceptable. The **American National Standards Institute (ANSI)**

American National Standards Institute (ANSI)

standards for the safe use of lasers in health care facilities.

Requirements	Safety Training and Education
ANSI Standards	Employ Laser Safety Officer
	Follow state and federal regulations for use
	Develop standards of care
	Assure safety to clients and staff
	Provide equipment safety and maintenance

© Milady, a part of Cengage Learning.

Figure 8–4 The American National Standards Institute (ANSI) safety requirements.

New lasers are now frequently being developed and sold with more advanced safety features. Always use the safety recommendations of the laser manufacturer, which include proper room design.

has created standards for the safe use of lasers in healthcare facilities (Figure 8–4). These standards are used by OSHA and every facility—no matter how small—must comply. Also established is a laser hazard classification that is used by the FDA and ANSI.

The design of the laser room is an important part of the safe use of lasers. The room should be set up with a well-grounded outlet, a separate circuit breaker, proper ventilation, nonreflective surfaces, either no windows or windows blocked with protective covering, and a door that can be locked during the service. Eye protection should be made available to those planning to enter the treatment room, and a danger sign should be posted on the exterior of the door (Figure 8–5).

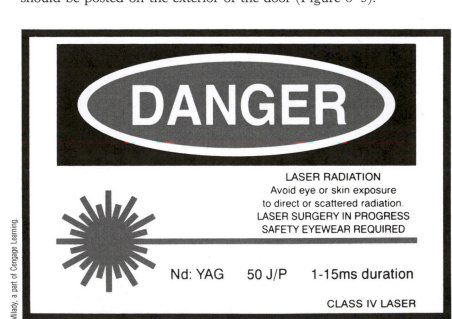

© Milady, a part of Cengage Learning.

Figure 8–5 A danger sign must be placed on the outside of the laser room door.

Nonablative Lasers

Nonablative lasers do not remove the skin; the laser light heats the dermis, leaving the epidermis intact. The treatments require multiple sessions, usually in a series every three to four weeks. Treatments can be painful and can require topical anesthesia and some pain medication. New technology is being released that creates minimal pain. Recovery time is minimal.

Uses of Nonablative Lasers

Nonablative lasers are used for the following conditions:

- **Vascular lesions**: Lasers destroy vascular lesions by targeting the oxyhemoglobin (red blood cells).
- **Pigmented lesions**: These are removed by targeting the melanin in the skin.
- Loss of elasticity: The increased heat wounds the dermal level.

vascular lesions
a rupture or malformation of blood vessels near the skin's surface. Common types include broken capillaries, spider veins, port wine stains, and hemanigomas.

pigmented lesions
melanin in the skin.

Types of Nonablative Lasers

Nonablative lasers can be intense pulsed light, pulsed dye, ND, and YAG (normal mode and long pulse mode). Refer to Figure 8–6 for a chart of lasers and the conditions indicated for their use.

Category of Laser	Used for	Types of Lasers Used
Ablative	Resurfacing, vascular lesions, pigmented lesions, loss of elasticity	Short and variable pulsed Erbium: YAG, Fractional lasers, CO_2 Laser, Titanyl Phosphate KTiOPO laser, (KTP), Argon, ND: YAG, Ruby QS, and Alexandrite QS
Nonablative	Vascular lesions, pigmented lesions, loss of elasticity	Intense Pulsed Light, Pulsed Dye, ND: YAG normal mode and long pulse
Hair Removal	Hair removal	Ruby, Alexandrite, Diode, ND: YAG normal mode, Intense Pulsed Light

© Milady, a part of Cengage Learning.

Figure 8–6 Categories and types of lasers used.

fractionated laser
utilizes the 1550 nm wavelength and targets water in the skin, which leaves the stratum corneum attached.

Fractional Resurfacing

A **fractionated laser** utilizes the 1550 nm wavelength and targets water in the skin, which leaves the stratum corneum attached. The laser beams are delivered in a randomized pattern, which creates columns of microscopic wounds within the dermis and epidermis. The healthy skin that surrounds the wounded tissue helps to accelerate the the wound healing process. **Fractional resurfacing is used to treat stage 1–2 aging conditions and hyperpigmentation.**

Results and Recovery

Fractional resurfacing treats moderate to severe wrinkles, acne scarring, and uneven skin texture. The skin may appear red and swollen for about three days after an aggressive treatment, which can be painful. In result, oral pain medication may be indicated. A less aggressive treatment will not be as painful and post-treatment inflammation will be less apparent. It can take up to six treatments to visibly improve the skin, and results can be seen slowly.

Intense Pulsed Light (IPL)

Intense pulsed light or IPL is a nonablative laser that uses a broad spectrum of light (non-coherent) instead of a single collimated beam at a specific wavelength. Intense pulsed light (IPL) can deliver multiple color combinations of light at a time. Pulsed light machines use cut-off filters to selectively deliver the desired wavelengths. These wavelengths can be customized to reach the specific hair, blood vessel, or skin component being treated and can be modified with each pulse.

Pulsed light begins with all wavelengths of light, from 500 to 1200 nm, including green, yellow, red, and infrared light. Various lower range, shorter wavelength (515 to 755 nm) cut-off filters block light shorter than the wavelength of the filter. Because longer wavelengths penetrate deeper into the target, longer wavelengths are used to treat deeper targets and to avoid and protect superficial parts of the skin. Shorter wavelengths are used to treat more superficial targets without damaging deeper areas of the skin.

Pulsed light can be delivered in pulses or bursts that vary from one to five pulses at a time. The duration of each pulse and the delay between pulses can be modified for each treatment site. Longer durations are generally better for treating larger targets, and shorter pulse durations are generally better for treating smaller areas.

IPL is used to treat stage 1 & 2 aging conditions, hyperpigmentation, and vascular conditions.

Results and Recovery

The results of IPL can include pigmented spots that may crust within five days, and mild erythema may be present for one week. However, there is minimal downtime with this type of treatment.

Photopneumatic Technology

Photopneumatic technology is essentially a vacuum combined with IPL. The gentle vacuum is specifically designed to gently pull the target chromophore toward the light source in the attachment. The vacuum reduces the diameter of the blood vessel within the skin as the IPL is administered. This decreases the amount of competing chromophores, which allows four to five times more photons to impact the target. This technique also reduces the amount of input energy lost to reflection, scatter, and absorption. The claim is that this makes the IPL treatment five times more effective, providing a painless treatment for pigmentation problems, varicose veins, and hair removal. **Photopneumatic technology is used to treat stage 1–2 aging conditions and hyperpigmentation.**

Results and Recovery

Results depend on the strength of the treatment, and multiple sessions may be required. Photopneumatic technology has the same recovery as an IPL treatment.

The Esthetician's Role

Fully understanding spot size, fluence, wavelength, thermal storage coefficient, pulse duration, and thermal relaxation time is important for the esthetician. Most lasers have preprogrammed parameters that eliminate guesswork, but it is still important to understand why the laser works the way it does.

For laser resurfacing, estheticians will mainly be involved with pre-treatment and post-treatment care depending on the state they are working in. A basic wound healing protocol will be designed by the physician, physician assistant, or registered nurse (RN) responsible for the treatment outcome. Following directions will be vital to avoid a liability situation, even with a non-invasive laser treatment. Of course, a well-trained esthetician can recognize when something needs to be corrected and should be able to communicate concerns to the person giving directions.

To create effective treatments, it is important to understand the wound-healing process, wound care, basic chemistry, cellular biology, and basic pharmaceuticals. For example, a client may be taking a **nonsteroidal anti-inflammatory drug (NSAID)** and the herb St. John's Wort,

nonsteroidal anti-inflammatory drug (NSAID)
medications used primarily to treat inflammation, mild to moderate pain, and fever.

either of which can impair wound healing. This information is included in the advanced clinical training available to estheticians post graduation or in a highly skilled primary training program.

Skin Tightening Technology

Radiofrequency

Radiofrequency (RF) technology uses electromagnetic radiation to heat up the dermal tissue, causing a wound process in the skin. RF is a form of electromagnetic energy between 30 kHz-300 GHz, skin treatments generally use between 3 MHz to 30 MHz. It is similar to lasers in that it creates a thermal change within the skin. Unlike lasers, RF does not target a chromophore; it is nonablative and generates heat through tissue resistance to the flow of electrons within the RF field. RF energy creates dermal heating to 149 degrees Fahrenheit.[1] This causes collagen to shrink, which causes sagging skin to tighten as the dermis begins to heal. Within the skin RF radiation will produce different thermal effects based on electrode configuration: monopolar RF will penetrate deeply into the dermis, but bipolar RF will provide only superficial penetration. Monopolar and bipolar RF are used together for more effective results, and RF is also combined with IPL to treat wrinkles and loss of elasticity. It has been found that the two technologies used together can have a better effect. **RF is used to treat stage 1–2 aging conditions.**

Results and Recovery

The results of RF are not immediate; it can take up to 12 weeks for the tightening effects to be visible. Radiofrequency is a painful treatment, and a mild sedative is given beforehand. Multiple treatments may be required.

The Esthetician's Role

Radiofrequency is a modality often performed by estheticians in a medical spa or clinic. Training is usually provided by the manufacturer or clinic before use, and it is important to follow the directions given. The goal with some skin tightening technology is to keep the heat within the skin as long as possible, which would negate the possibility of a cooling soothing facial treatment after application.

Dermal Fillers

Dermal fillers or soft tissue augmentation were first developed in 1893 by F. Nueber, who transplanted fat from the arms of patients to improve defects. Silicone was then used in the middle 20th century until it was banned in 1992. Since then a new form was developed and approved for use by the FDA. Dermal fillers are used to treat lines, wrinkles, and loss of skin density. There are currently several dermal fillers on the market, with many more being considered, which can be classified as temporary fillers, semi-permanent fillers, and permanent fillers.

Temporary Fillers

Temporary fillers are designed to last from 4 to 12 months and are biodegradable. Temporary fillers are usually the first step in fillers, so that the patient can determine if the results meet expectations. They are used for superficial-to-deep lines and wrinkles, loss of skin density, and scarring throughout the face. **Temporary fillers are used to treat stage 2–3 aging conditions (no skin texture improvement).**

Contraindications for dermal fillers of all types are: autoimmune diseases, inflammatory disorders, allergic history, history of **anaphylactic** reactions, pregnant or breastfeeding, and undergoing immunosuppressant therapy. Hylaform Plus cannot be used by patients allergic to eggs.

The temporary dermal fillers available are outlined in the sections that follow.

anaphylactic
rapidly developing and serious allergic reaction that affects a number of different areas of the body at one time

Collagen

Bovine collagen (Zyderm, Zyplast), bioengineered skin collagen (CosmoDerm, CosmoPlast). Duration is about four months.

- **Benefits:** treats deep wrinkles and scars, appropriate for the vermillion border (Zyplast), superficial lines, horizontal forehead wrinkles, crow's feet, fine perioral wrinkles (Zyderm). Can be safely reinjected three to four times a year. Contains .3 percent lidocaine to reduce pain. Collagen has a lower cost than other dermal fillers.
- Bioengineered collagen is non-allergenic and is used to treat medium to deep wrinkles. It is associated with less bruising and contains lidocaine to reduce pain. HA fillers can be used with bioengineered collagen to treat superficial lines and deep lines at the same time.
- **Cautions:** approximately 3 percent of population is allergic to bovine collagen and it should not be used on people with a history of autoimmune disease. Patients must be tested for allergy before injection. Side effects can include abscesses, bacterial infections, beading, cysts, granuloma formation, and skin death in area of injection. Bioengineered collagen is more expensive but has the same possible side effects except the allergic reaction.

Hyaluronic Acid

Animal derived (Hylaform Plus), bacterial derived (Restylane®, Juvéderm®, Perlane®). Duration is about 6–12 months.

- **Benefits:** longer duration than collagen, nonallergenic, does not require prior testing, fewer side effects.
- **Cautions:** side effects are mild and can include swelling, bruising, lumps, and acne eruptions. Vascular problems rarely occur around injection site. Increased pain, edema, and erythema are common, and an anesthetic should be used.

The Esthetician's Role

The use of fillers is gaining in popularity and certainly will be a treatment alternative brought up by the aging client. Knowing all the facts about dermal fillers will be important, which includes contraindications and post care. Advising the client about good home care to help prevent further aging is important.

Treatment guidelines are:

- No manipulation of the injection area for at least 48–72 hours after injection (for safety), which means no facial right after injection.
- No UV exposure for three to five days.
- No alcohol for at least six hours.
- Exercise allowed after six hours.
- No prolonged ice application for 24 hours.
- Reduce facial expressions for six to eight hours.
- A hydrating facial has been used in the medical spa to enhance the effects of the dermal filler.

Dermal fillers are often combined with Botulinum Toxin Type A with good results when done by an experienced injector. This is often marketed as the *liquid face-lift*. Dermal fillers that are commonly used with Botulinum Toxin are: Restylane, Hylaform, Hylaform 2, Cosmo-Derm, and CosmoPlast.[2]

Botulinum Toxin Type A

Botulinum Toxin (Botox) was first used for cosmetic purposes in 1981 and was approved for treatment of frown lines (glabellar lines) by the FDA in 2002. It is considered one of the most popular non-invasive anti-aging therapies available today. Botulinum Toxin works by stopping acetylcholine from stimulating the nerves at the neuromuscular junction, which stops the muscle from receiving the signal to move, thus causing paralysis of the muscle (Figure 8–7). **Botulinum Toxin**

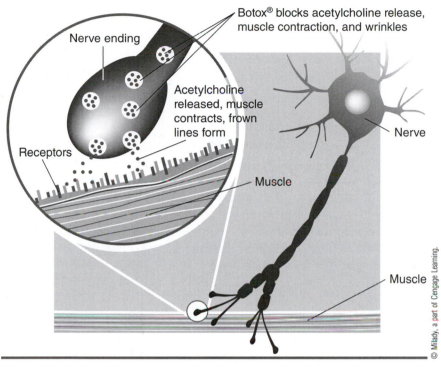

Botox® blocks acetylcholine release, muscle contraction, and wrinkles

Nerve ending

Acetylcholine released, muscle contracts, frown lines form

Receptors

Nerve

Muscle

Muscle

© Milady, a part of Cengage Learning.

Figure 8–7 Botox® has a highly complex process of action.

Type A is used to treat stage 1–2 aging conditions (dynamic expression and static rhytids, no texture improvement).

Two types of Botulinum Toxin have been approved by the FDA for cosmetic use:

- **Botox:** produced by Allergan, first approved in the United States in 2002, lasts approximately three to five months, takes three to five days to work with full effects seen at 14 days.
- **Dysport/Reloxin:** produced by Medicis, approved for use in the United States in 2009, lasts six months to one year, takes one to three days to see effects. The cost per dose is less than Botox but more units will have to be used to achieve the same effects.[3]

Contraindications and Side Effects

Botulinum Toxin is not to be used if the following contraindications are present:

- Hypersensitivity to Botulinum Toxin
- Infection
- Neuromuscular disorders

- Autoimmune disorders
- Pregnancy or breast feeding
- Under anesthesia
- Body dysmorphic disorder

Side effects can be:

- Headache
- Bruising at site of injection
- Eye or brow ptosis (Figure 8–8)
- Development of neutralizing antibodies
- Asymmetry after injection
- Possible migration from injection site: Recently there was a study released causing controversy over the fact that Botulinum Toxin was seen to migrate from the point of injection to the nervous system of rats, suggesting that the same may be possible in humans.[4]

In 2009 the FDA approved a new insert for Botox which provides in-depth information on the side effects and interactions that can happen upon injection.

The Esthetician's Role

Estheticians should understand the basics and contraindications of Botulinum Toxin to answer client questions (Figure 8–9). Advising the client about good home care to help prevent further aging is important.

Treatment guidelines are:

- No manipulation of the injection area for at least 72 hours after injection (for safety), which means no facial right after injection.
- A hydrating facial treatment before injection can be helpful.

> It is important that estheticians understand the new Botox® label, because this is not given out by most medical practitioners before a Botox injection. The label comes with the vials on purchase, which are then used as needed, for multiple clients. Thorough informed consent should cover this information.

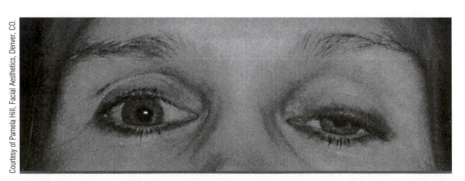

Courtesy of Pamela Hill, Facial Aesthetics, Denver, CO.

Figure 8–8 When the injection is close to the eyebrow, an eyelid ptosis may occur.

Medication Guide

Botox® may cause serious side effects that can be life threatening. Call your doctor or get medical help right away if you have any of these problems after treatment with Botox:

- **Problems swallowing, speaking, or breathing.** These problems can happen hours to weeks after an injection of Botox® usually because the muscles that you use to breathe and swallow can become weak after the injection. Death can occur as a complication if you have severe problems with swallowing or breathing after treatment with Botox®.
- People with certain breathing problems may need to use muscles in their necks to help them breathe. These patients may be at greater risk for serious breathing problems with Botox®.
- Swallowing problems may last for several months. People who cannot swallow well may need a feeding tube to receive food and water. If swallowing problems are severe, food or liquids may go into your lungs. People who already have swallowing or breathing problems before receiving **BOTOX®** or **BOTOX®** Cosmetic have the highest risk of experiencing these problems.
- **Spread of toxin effects.** In some cases, the effect of botulinum toxin may affect areas of the body away from the injection site and cause symptoms of a serious condition called botulism. The symptoms of botulism include:

  - Loss of strength and muscle weakness all over the body
  - Double vision
  - Blurred vision and drooping eyelids
  - Hoarseness or change or loss of voice (dysphonia)
  - Trouble saying words clearly (dysarthria)
  - Loss of bladder control
  - Trouble breathing
  - Trouble swallowing

These symptoms can happen hours to weeks after you receive an injection.

Source: Botox Medication Guide from the Food and Drug Administration.

Cell Therapy

Cell therapy is a new type of non-invasive anti-aging treatment that extracts fibroblasts from the patient's skin, causes them to multiply into millions of new cells, freezes them then reinjects cells back into the patient's skin. This is proposed to increase the skin's ability to

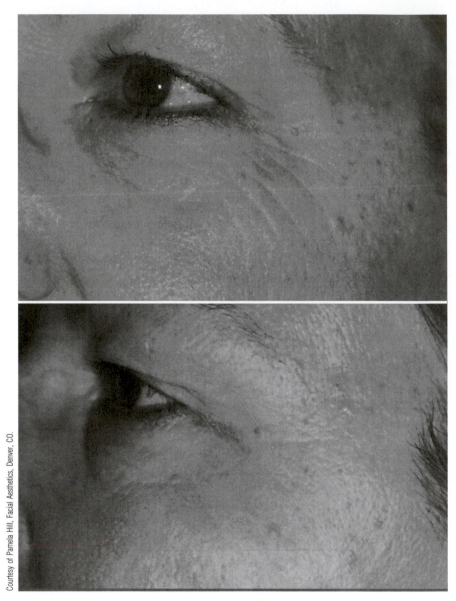

Courtesy of Pamela Hill, Facial Aesthetics, Denver, CO.

Figure 8–9 Before and after treatment with Botox at the crow's feet.

create collagen. The trade name for this procedure is Laviv. The procedure is currently undergoing testing by the FDA for approval for treatment of moderate to severe nasolabial folds. **Cell therapy is used to treat stage 2–3 aging conditions.**

The Esthetician's Role

It is unknown at this time what the role of esthetician will be; it is safe to say that basic skin health advice and treatments will need to be done to keep the client's skin in good health and protect it from further damage.

Medium and Deep Peels

Chemical peels have been one of the most popular cosmetic procedures in the aesthetic medical market for many years. Many estheticians perform medium-depth peels under medical supervision. **Peels are used to treat stage 1–3 aging conditions and hyperpigmentation in lighter Fitzpatrick types.**

There are several options for medical-level peels:

- **Resorcinol**: used since 1882.[5] Not to be used on darker Fitzpatrick types. Resorcinol can cause contact dermatitis. Peeling occurs over seven days and irritation. Used for acne and pigment disorders.[6]
- **Jessner's Peel**: this solution is 14 g salicylic acid, 14 g resorcinol, and 14 g lactic acid in an ethanol base. The strength of the peel is determined by the layers applied to the skin and is self-neutralizing. Modified Jessner's are commonly used with other acids, which include hydroquinone and kojic acid for treatment of hyperpigmentation. Jessner's peel is not intended for darker Fitzpatrick types. Peeling occurs over 7–10 days depending on the number of layers applied.[7]
- **TCA**: trichloroacetic acid is used in strengths of 10–40 percent. Lower percentages are used to treat fine lines and wrinkles. Higher percentages cause dermal and epidermal necrosis, which treats deeper wrinkles and pigmentation disorders. Scarring can occur. Can be used on darker Fitzpatrick types with careful pretreatment prepping. It can be layered with a Jessner's peel or glycolic acid for a deeper peel and healing time can be from 5–10 days depending on the layers used.
- **Pyruvic Acid**: penetrates to the papillary dermis, which stimulates collagen and elastin formation. Pyruvic acid has a high potential for scarring. Not for use on darker Fitzpatrick types, sensitive skin, or irritated skin. To reduce client discomfort, the peel will be neutralized with baking soda and water. The peel must be done in a well-ventilated room due to the fumes. Healing time is one to two weeks, with erythema possibly lasting up to two months.[8]

The Esthetician's Role

Post-treatment care is vitally important with medium and deep peels. The client will experience discomfort and extensive flaking and peeling. Post-care is important.

Post-treatment guidelines are:

- Avoid UV exposure for at least one week; use a broad spectrum block daily, preferably a physical block such as zinc oxide. A double application of sunscreen is recommended while healing.
- Avoid removing any peeling areas of face.
- Use a gentle nonsurfactant cleanser; do not exfoliate until area is completely healed.
- Use an emollient as needed, keeping the skin moist consistently.
- If allowed by supervising medical personnel, a mild enzyme peel approximately a week after the treatment will help with the peeling phase.

> The esthetician's role in medical aesthetics is as much an art as it is a science. Doctors are finding new beneficial ways to perform treatments that may change the currently accepted models. The main point to remember is that an esthetician should take guidance from the physician and realize that the information presented here are general guidelines. Always remember your state's scope of practice as well.

■ OPTIONS FOR INVASIVE TREATMENT

Invasive treatments refer to treatments that remove tissue, require an extended healing period, and require medication to manage pain during the treatment as well as post-treatment. This category includes cosmetic surgery. The esthetician's role will be limited until a specific period of healing time has passed.

Ablative Lasers

Ablative lasers are lasers that ablate, or remove, skin. The laser light is absorbed by the water, oxyhemoglobin, and melanin within the skin to accomplish this task. The more tissue to be removed, the higher the energy used and the more passes performed during treatment. The treatment is painful and requires topical anesthesia and some pain medication. Recovery time could last from a few days to a week or more.

Use of Ablative Lasers

Ablative lasers are used for the following reasons:

- Resurfacing (texture and wrinkling): Resurfacing is accomplished by targeting the water in the skin.
- Vascular lesions: Lasers destroy vascular lesions by targeting the oxyhemoglobin (red blood cells).

- Pigmented lesions: These are removed by the laser targeting the melanin in the skin.
- Loss of elasticity: This is treated with increased heat to target the dermal level.

Types of Ablative Lasers

The following types of ablative lasers are used in treatment:

- Short and variable-pulsed erbium: YAG (yttrium aluminum garnet)
- Fractional
- CO_2
- Titanyl phosphate (KTiOPO) lasers, also called KTP lasers
- Argon
- ND YAG (neodymium-doped yttrium aluminum garnet; $Nd:Y_3Al_5O_{12}$) ruby QS
- Alexandrite QS

Ablative Fractional Resurfacing: An ablative fractionated laser creates micro-columns of heat-induced injury with coagulation, ablation, and thermal stimulation of the dermis with proprietary wavelengths that targets water in the skin. This leaves the stratum corneum attached as the laser beams are delivered in a randomized pattern, which creates columns of microscopic wounds within the dermis and epidermis. The healthy skin that surrounds the wounded tissue accelerates the wound healing process.

Ablative Fractional Resurfacing Treatments: Ablative fractional resurfacing treats moderate to severe wrinkles, acne scarring, and uneven skin texture and loss of firmness. **Ablative fractional resurfacing treats stage 2–3 aging conditions, hyper-/hypopigmentation, and vascular conditions.**

Risks and Recovery: The skin may appear red and swollen for about three days after an aggressive treatment, which can be painful; oral pain medication may be indicated. A less aggressive treatment will not be as painful, and post-treatment inflammation will be less apparent. It can take up to six treatments to visibly improve the skin, and results can be seen slowly.

Plasma

Plasma is inert nitrogen gas that is delivered into the skin. The skin starts to shed much like a chemical peel within a few days after application. The depth of treatment depends on the number of passes

General surgical guidelines for cosmetic surgery on the face include the following:

- Do not smoke for four to six weeks before or after surgery.
- Do not take vitamin E, herbs, aspirin or aspirin products, or any other supplement unless the doctor approves.
- Only take medication approved by the doctor.
- Follow post-surgery diet of clear liquids; stop all liquids by 12:00 am the night before surgery.
- Wear loose-fitting clothing.
- Sleep elevated on back.
- Do not shower for 24 hours.
- Limit sexual activities.
- Avoid exercise until instructed by doctor.

performed. Treatment is generally well tolerated except for more aggressive treatments that require multiple passes.

Plasma Treatments: This technology is used to treat fine to moderate wrinkles, pigmentation problems, skin lesions, and to tighten skin. **Plasma treats stage 2–3 aging conditions.**

Risks and Recovery: Aggressive treatment requires topical anesthetic, oral sedatives, and may take multiple treatments; results are generally seen in 10 days.

Cosmetic Surgery

Eye Lift

Known as blepharoplasty, surgery used to correct aging eye issues such as sagging lids, puffiness under eyes, to tighten lower eye, and to reposition upper or lower eyelid (Figure 8–10). **Eye lift treats stage 2–3 aging conditions around eyes.**

Risks and Recovery

The possible complications with blepharoplasty are bleeding, scarring, infection, cornea scratches, poor aesthetic results, and inability to close eyes. Recovery varies based on patient health; stitches are removed in three to five days and bruising can last up to a month. In addition to normal surgical guidelines, post-care guidelines are:

- Keep head elevated.
- Use cold compresses.
- Gently clean eyes with distilled water to remove discharge from wounds.
- Use eye drops as needed for dryness.
- Use sunglasses and avoid the sun.
- Do not use contact lenses.
- Limit reading, watching TV, or working on the computer to avoid eye strain.

Face-Lift

Face-lifts are called rhytidectomy. Cosmetic surgeons use several techniques. The traditional rhytidectomy does not involve the upper portion of the face, and a forehead and brow lift can be combined with this procedure. This procedure is indicated for loss of firmness, deep nasolabial folds, and wrinkles in lower portion of face and neck,

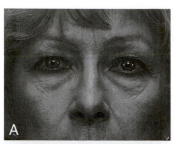
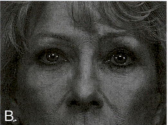
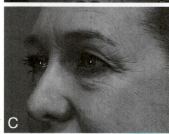
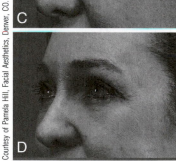

Courtesy of Pamela Hill, Facial Aesthetics, Denver, CO.

Figure 8–10 (a) Before blepharoplasty. (b) After blepharoplasty. (c) Before four-lid blepharoplasty. (d) After four-lid blepharoplasty.

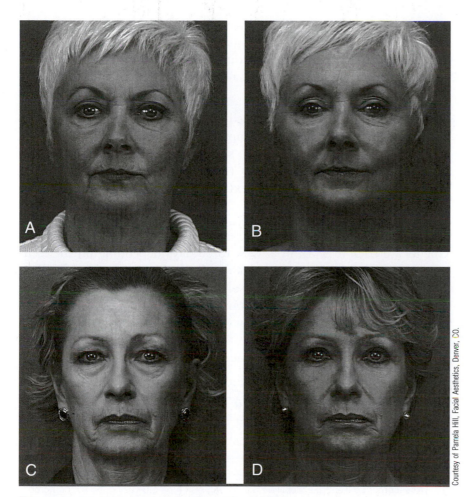

Courtesy of Pamela Hill, Facial Aesthetics, Denver, CO.

Figure 8–11 Before and after face-lift patients.

sagging jawline, fatty neck, and neck cords. Figure 8–11 shows an example of the before and after photos of a face-lift. This procedure is usually performed under general anesthesia; physicians have their own preference based on techniques used.

Face-lifts are used to treat stage 3 aging conditions on lower face and neck (except for texture and pigmentation issues).

Risks and Recovery

Edema occurs within 24–48 hours after surgery and can last several weeks. Scarring is minimal unless a darker Fitzpatrick type; then keloid scarring could be possible. Numbness will be present over several months and could be permanent. Healing is gradual and full results will not be seen for several months. Clients can return to work within one week. Follow general surgical guidelines for recovery.

Risks include: hematoma, bleeding, infection, hair loss around incision, injuries to sensory or motor nerves, reactions to anesthesia, and skin necrosis (smokers).

- **Forehead and Brow Lift:** used to treat the upper part of the face; not included in a face-lift. Improves forehead wrinkles (dynamic expression rhytides), raises a sagging eye, and smoothes frown lines (Figure 8–12). **Used to treat stage 2–3 aging conditions on upper face (except for texture, pigmentation).**

Risks and Recovery:

Clients are back to work in a week to 10 days depending on the technique used. Endoscopic techniques require less recovery time. Swelling and bruising occur and usually resolve in seven to nine days.

Risks include: bleeding, infection, hair loss along scar edges, sensory loss along incision line, loss of ability to raise eyebrows and forehead.

Now let's look at options for our case study.

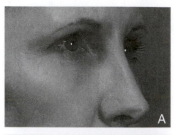
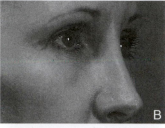
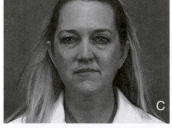
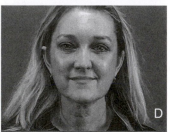

Courtesy of Pamela Hill, Facial Aesthetics, Denver, CO.

Figure 8–12 Before and after face-lift patients.

Case Study

Client: 42-year-old female

Skin type: Combination-Fitzpatrick Type 2

Conditions: Photodamage (hyperpigmentation), fine lines (stage 1 aging), dehydration, hyperkeratinized (dead skin cell buildup), comedones (blackheads)

Assessment: Client has identified with wrong skin type thus using the wrong home care products, high stress levels are impacting hydration and texture issues in the skin. Perimenopausal symptoms are adding to skin condition. Fitzpatrick type is good for most clinical treatments.

Goal: Increase desquamation to reduce fine lines, increase fibroblast stimulation, hydration (free water in the epidermis), increase microcirculation and lymphatic flow (oxygenation of the skin), exfoliate the stratum corneum, suppress melanin production (inhibit tyrosinase production, reduce melanosome transfer), reduce inflammation, increase free radical protection, and induce the relaxation response in the body.

Medical treatment options: Botox injections, IPL for pigmentation issues, and fractionated laser treatments.

The esthetician's role: Get skin into healthy balanced state through treatments and effective home care. Provide education on how important it is to protect skin and soothe, calm, and hydrate skin after treatments to prevent long-term damage.

These procedures are just some of the techniques used to treat aging skin at an aesthetic medical office. New techniques and technologies are being developed all the time. It is important for estheticians to continue to research and learn what is being done through trade journals, trade shows, and advanced education. What an exciting time to be an esthetician with so much to learn!

> > > **Top Ten Tips to Take to the Clinic**

1. Know your state's scope of practice.
2. Understand the basic physics of light.
3. Know the difference between ablative and nonablative treatments.
4. Understand the wound healing process when working with clients who have undergone medical treatment.
5. Understand an esthetician's role in medical treatments.
6. Educate your client about appropriate post-care.
7. Understand the possible side effects and complications of aesthetic medical treatments.
8. Understand the different treatments available for the client based on their goals and concerns.
9. Understand the safety requirements when working with lasers.
10. Know the different types of chemical peels and how they work on the skin.

Chapter Review Questions

1. What does LASER stand for?
2. What are ANSI standards?
3. How long should you wait before doing a facial treatment on a client who has had a Botox injection?
4. What is cell therapy and what is the proposed benefit of this treatment?
5. What is the esthetician's role in aesthetic medical treatments?

References

1. Schmaling, S. (2008). *Milady's Aesthetician Series: A Comprehensive Guide to Equipment*. Clifton Park, NY: Cengage Learning.
2. Hill, P. (2006). Milady's Aesthetician Series: Botox, Dermal Fillers, and Sclerotherapy. Clifton Park, NY: Delmar Learning.
3. Schmaling, S. (2008). *Milady's Aesthetician Series: A Comprehensive Guide to Equipment*. Clifton Park, NY: Cengage Learning.
4. Antonucci, F., et al. (2008). "Long-Distance Retrograde Effects of Botulinum Neurotoxin A." *The Journal of Neuroscience*, 28 (14): 3689–3696.

5. Baumann, L. MD., Saghari, S. MD., Weisburg, E. MS. (2009). *Cosmetic Dermatology: Principles and Practice*, 2nd Edition. New York: McGraw Hill.
6. Baumann, L. MD., Saghari, S. MD., Weisburg, E. MS. (2009). *Cosmetic Dermatology: Principles and Practice*, 2nd Edition. New York: McGraw Hill.
7. Baumann, L. MD., Saghari, S. MD., Weisburg, E. MS. (2009). *Cosmetic Dermatology: Principles and Practice*, 2nd Edition. New York: McGraw Hill.
8. Baumann, L. MD., Saghari, S. MD., Weisburg, E. MS. (2009). *Cosmetic Dermatology: Principles and Practice*, 2nd Edition. New York: McGraw Hill.

Bibliography

Arroyave, E. MD. (2006). *Understanding Cosmetic Procedures: Surgical and Nonsurgical*. Clifton Park, NY: Cengage Learning.
Hill, P., Pickart, M. MD. (2009). *Milady's Aesthetician Series: Cosmetic Surgery and the Aesthetician*. Clifton Park, NY: Cengage Learning.

Websites

Botox medication guide from the Food and Drug Administration:
www.fda.gov/downloads/Drugs/DrugSafety/UCM176360.pdf
www.fibrocell.com

Lifestyle Choices

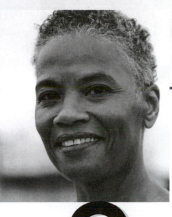

chronic obstructive
   pulmonary disease
   (COPD)

dopamine receptors
excoriations
stress

THC (delta-9-
   tetrahydro-
   cannabinol)
zazen

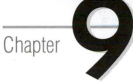

Chapter **9**

After completing this chapter, you will be able to:

1. Discuss lifestyle choices and their effects on skin.
2. Identify options for treatment.
3. Describe drug use and its effects on skin.

■ INTRODUCTION

A client's lifestyle choices can have profound effects on aging and are the one thing that the client has full control over. Estheticians can provide information about healthy lifestyle choices to clients, but it is not within the esthetic code of ethics to judge or coerce lifestyle choices.

However, it is important to be completely honest with clients about how the choices they make will affect the outcome of treatments. For example, trying to improve the appearance of aging in the skin of smokers is difficult, if not impossible, and the client needs to understand this. In this chapter we review many of the common lifestyle choices that can impact a healthy aging plan.

■ THE EFFECTS OF STRESS

stress
term commonly used to describe a physical and mental response to stressors.

Chronic stress can be one of the most destructive processes in the body. It is the one lifestyle condition that the esthetician has a positive impact on. Understanding how stress impacts the body is important when designing a healthy aging program.

Stress is a term commonly used to describe a physical and mental response to stressors. Stressors can be physical, such as injury or illness, or they can be psychological, such as death of a spouse, financial trouble, or moving.

The stress response within the body is a complex set of actions that are interdependent. A reaction to stress starts with *fight or flight* response. This is a surge of adrenaline and cortisol within the body that increases blood flow to the muscles. Breathing quickens, blood pressure rises, and senses become more acute. When this process is working properly it can help focus, stamina, and performance.

The longer this stress response is *on* the harder it is for it to stop and the easier it becomes for the stress response to be activated. This is the cycle of chronic stress which can lead to problems such as cardiovascular disease, type II diabetes, headaches, ulcers, and autoimmune diseases. In addition, a link has been verified between chronic stress and premature aging by the shortening of telomeres. See Chapter 4 for information on aging theories.

The causes of chronic stress are as varied as people (Figure 9–1). Some situations are universally considered to produce negative stress:

- Death of a loved one
- Financial problems

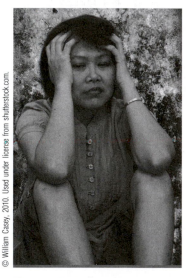

Figure 9–1 Chronic stress can be one of the most destructive processes in the body.

Quick Stress Busters

Stop and breathe. Take a deep breath in to the count of 5, and exhale as you count to 5. Do this 10 times.

Laugh. Rent a funny movie, watch comedy shows, or call a funny friend.

Find a visual focus. Pick a beautiful scene to watch, or focus on mundane things such as counting people with red shirts. Do that for at least one minute.

Spray an aromatherapy stress blend in your space and inhale. A good blend is: 6 ounces of distilled water, 15 drops of lavender, 6–8 drops of orange, and 2 drops of cinnamon. Shake then spray. Use your senses; the aromatherapy that appeals to you is what you need.

Move. Walk, stretch, and run if needed for at least five minutes. This is in addition to regular exercise needed daily.

- Relationship problems
- Chronic pain

Other situations are open to interpretation and perception. For example, speaking in front of a large group is terrifying for some and exhilarating for others. The physical response is the same but managing that response is different. Good coping skills and a healthy positive outlook are key.

The physical symptoms of chronic stress are important to recognize in order to provide the right treatment and advice. They are:

- Biting nails
- Shallow breathing
- Quick movements
- Fast speaking
- Fidgeting
- Sighing
- Darting eyes
- Frequent touching of face and hair
- Rubbing eyes
- Negative self-comments
- General look of sadness
- Looking tired

These are all symptoms to be aware of in order to start the dialogue about how the client is feeling and what stressors may be affecting

Stress that is perceived as psychological is just as harmful as a physical stressor and should not be dismissed with a comment such as *It's all in your head*. Several studies have found a direct physical response to psychological stress.

them. Some of the physical symptoms that the client may be experiencing that cannot be seen are:

- Insomnia (sleep disorders can start with stress or contribute to it)
- Lack of appetite
- Increased appetite, especially for sugary, fatty foods
- Negative self-talk
- Lack of concentration
- Confusion, impaired decision-making
- Depression
- Anxiety
- Chest pain
- Dizziness
- Loss of libido
- Increased illnesses
- Headaches
- Psychological symptoms that the client may be experiencing
- Using alcohol, cigarettes, and drugs for relief (self-medicating)
- Procrastinating or neglecting responsibilities
- Isolating themselves from contact with others
- Moodiness
- Anger
- Sensory overload (sights, sounds, and even smells can agitate)

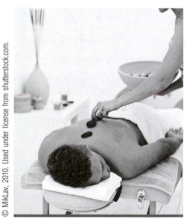

© MikLav, 2010. Used under license from shutterstock.com.

Figure 9–2 Massage incorporates both psychological and physical relief.

HOW TO MANAGE STRESS

Stress will occur, and there will be periods in a person's life when stress feels constant and out of control. Coping strategies are important to learn, and different modalities that can help are briefly explained in the sections that follow.

Massage

The esthetician knows the importance of massage, and it should be included regularly when dealing with high levels of stress (Figure 9–2). See Chapter 6 for detailed information on massage. The type of massage used for stress reduction is a gentle stimulation massage. This type of massage provides a temporary diversion to the nervous system, which can shut down the fight or flight response and give the client a chance to regroup. The reactions that a client will have are two-fold:

- **Psychological**: touch helps relieve anxiety, fear, and loneliness.
- **Physical**: adrenal secretions slow down, breathing slows and deepens, pulse slows down, blood pressure lowers, and feel-good hormones such as oxytocin are released in the body. For chronic pain, massage can divert attention from the acute pain and increase oxygen and nutrients to the area while removing lactic acid.

Meditation

The practice of meditation has long been a part of spiritual practices but is now being implemented into secular health management. The benefits of meditation have been widely documented and should be looked at as a stress reduction technique regardless of religious belief systems.

Meditation induces the relaxation response within the body. This response lowers heart rate, reduces cortisol production, slows respiration, lowers blood pressure, and changes brain chemisty.[1] Meditation has also been shown to influence an increase in gray matter within the parts of the brain that relate to attention and sensory input. It also has been theorized to help slow down deterioration associated with aging.[2]

Zen meditation is called **zazen**, and is one of the most common types of meditation. Counting breaths meditation is one that a beginner can start with 5 minutes a day, working up to twice a day for 30–45 minutes.

Healthy Sleep

Healthy sleep is vitally important for health and has direct effects on the stress response within the body (Figure 9–4). When the body is under chronic stress, insomnia is a common symptom. This lack of sleep affects learning, memory, mood, cardiovascular health, and hormones. It also affects the immune system by influencing cytokines responsible for inflammation. Chronically stressed, sleep-deprived individuals are more likely to develop infections as well.

Getting healthy sleep during a bout of chronic stress is a challenge. Here is some simple advice that the esthetician can give to the client:

- Get the right amount of sleep. The average adult needs at least seven hours of sleep, and some need up to nine. There is no evidence

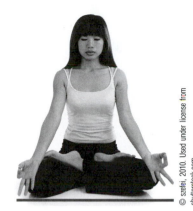

Figure 9–3 Meditation is a valuable stress reduction technique, with multiple benefits to the body.

Zazen
one of the most common types of meditation.

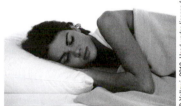

Figure 9–4 Healthy sleep is vital to good health and has direct effects on the stress response within the body.

Selling sleep aids such as eye pillows, aromatherapy sprays, and bath salts can be additional revenue but more importantly help your client through a hard situation (Figure 9–5).

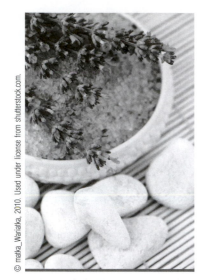

© matka_Wariatka, 2010. Used under license from shutterstock.com.

Figure 9–5 Aromatherapy sprays and bath salts can help to relax for better sleep.

Our emotional health shows up in our skin. Here are the signs:

● Oily shine: stress triggers the sebaceous glands to produce more.

● Skin conditions are aggravated: clients with rosacea, eczema, psoriasis will experience flares more frequently.

● Dull gray appearance: the stress response reduces blood flow to the surface of the skin.

that adults require less sleep when older, but rather that their biological clock shifts, and they spend less time in deep uninterrupted sleep.

- Keep to a sleep schedule. Consistently going to bed and waking at the same time, even on days off, will help.
- Exercise late in the day. Ideally, working out four to five hours before bed is needed to avoid overstimulation. That is not always possible, so follow the relaxation tips listed.
- Avoid alcohol before bed. Alcohol can make you sleepy but does not allow you to get deep rest.
- Avoid caffeine before bed. An evening cup of coffee or soda can be too stimulating.
- Set up your sleep space for sleep. Take out TVs and computers; use soothing colors, soft music, comfortable bedding as well as aromatherapy to induce relaxation.
- Take a bath. Hydrotherapy has system-wide benefits especially when incorporating aromatherapy, Epsom salts, seaweed, and mud.
- Avoid large meals right before bed. Digestion slows and a large meal can interfere with falling asleep.

Healthy Diet

A healthy diet is important when dealing with chronic stress. Small meals eaten at two- to three-hour intervals help maintain blood sugar levels and are easier on digestion. When a person is under stress, digestion slows considerably. A high complex carbohydrate, low protein diet is associated with reducing levels of cortisol, which is a major factor in the stress response.

The stress response also depletes antioxidants such as vitamin C and increases cravings of unhealthy foods, so supplementation is highly recommended. Several recommendations are:

- Beta carotene: this provitamin is essential for vitamin A creation.
- Vitamin B: complex B vitamins are essential for synthesis of prostaglandin hormones.
- Vitamin E: antioxidant vital to skin health and body function.
- Vitamin C: helps immune system and affects regulation of circulating cortisol and thyroid hormones.
- Zinc and magnesium: help with healthy adrenal glands and promote relaxation.
- Essential fatty acids: anti-inflammatory and support the skin.

See Chapter 10 for additional nutritional information.

Fitness

Fitness is essential to managing stress. Tai Chi is one of the most effective forms of exercise for stress and can act as a *moving meditation*. Yoga is another modality that can induce the relaxation response while strengthening muscles and increasing flexibility (Figure 9–6). See Chapter 11 for more fitness information.

Self-care

In this busy culture, self-care is often overlooked. Self-care encompasses both emotional and physical care. Esthetic treatments, massage, healthy sleep, and fitness can all be considered physical self-care. Emotional self-care is just as important but seems to be difficult for many chronically stressed clients. Here are some examples of emotional self-care that the esthetician can instruct the client on:

Change the situation; some stressors are out of a client's control, and others can be changed. Sometimes something as simple as changing the time of day that they leave for work to avoid heavy traffic can relieve tremendous stress. Here are other stress reducers:

- **Learning to say "No" when overwhelmed is valuable.**
- **Limit time spent with negative people.** If the client works with the public, using active listening skills can diffuse a negative situation. Learning that people are responsible for their own emotions is important for a stressed client. Many are caretakers and tuned into others' emotions and responses, which can be detrimental.
- **Manage personal environment.** Have a clean uncluttered space; avoid places that are noisy and aggravating; change time of day for commute and use extra time for meditation or walks.
- **Change the personal response.** This is the one thing a client can do to manage stress. Many emotional reactions are based on the perception that a person has about a situation. Changing the personal response or interpretation of the situation is one of the most effective ways to address stress.
- **Learn to forgive.** This is something that may require the help of a therapist if the issue to forgive is life altering. Accepting one's own mistakes is the first step in accepting the mistakes of others. Self-blaming can be a stress-inducing process.
- **Look for the positive in the situation.** There is always light after dark, and positive in a negative situation. Learning from mistakes and life lessons strengthens a person's resilience, which is a vital portion of a long healthy life.

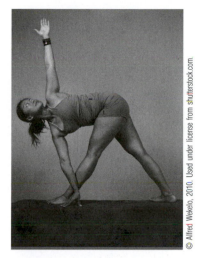

© Alfred Wekelo, 2010. Used under license from shutterstock.com.

Figure 9–6 Fitness is essential to managing stress. Yoga is a method to both relax and strengthen the body.

- **Look at situations with perspective.** Is the stressor as important now as it will be in the future?
- **Look at the facts objectively without emotion.** For example, "I have no money" is an emotional statement. "I have $2 in my bank account" is a fact. Facts may not be pleasant, but they are easier to deal with than emotions, and can lead to change.
- **Express feelings.** Feelings not expressed turn to resentment, which creates more stress.
- **Rely on personal spiritual practice.** A personal spiritual practice can give strength and comfort. Estheticians should be sensitive to these personal practices but refrain from trying to impose their beliefs on a client. Do not bring up issues of religion in the treatment room.
- **Learn to manage time.** Being organized and looking realistically at how to manage time are excellent ways to approach stress. There are many resources available from which clients can learn organizational skills.
- **Learn to be more assertive.** This falls in line with expressing feelings. Understanding personal boundaries and expressing them is important. This is an area where an esthetician can help the client. Instructing clients on how to express their needs during a service can help them start to be more assertive.
- **Do not try to control an uncontrollable situation.** Accepting things that cannot be changed is hard but necessary. If the client's situation involves grief and loss, it is important to direct the client to professional help. Refer to the team of professionals assembled for healthy aging treatment in Chapter 3.

■ SMOKING AND THE SKIN

Smoking is one of the most common habits that have been implicated in external aging, along with sun exposure, drinking, and poor nutrition. Smoking cigarettes is associated with diseases such as emphysema, lung cancer, heart disease, **chronic obstructive pulmonary disease (COPD)** and chronic bronchitis. Smoking has been associated with the following symptoms within the skin:[3]

- Increased wrinkling
- Red or orange complexion
- Ashy pale coloring
- Puffiness

chronic obstructive pulmonary disease (COPD)
a progressive disease that makes it hard to breathe.

- Gauntness and loss of elasticity
- Yellow, irregularly thickened skin
- Increased pre-cancerous lesions

Cigarette smoke contains over 1,500 chemical ingredients, and smoking depletes the levels of vitamins C and E, which affect the skin's function as follows:

- Thinning the stratum corneum
- Increasing the action of MMPs
- Reducing vitamin A levels
- Reducing capillary and arterial blood flow, which in turn reduces nutrition and oxygen to cells as well as producing toxic waste product buildup
- Slowing wound healing

Clients who smoke can be successfully treated, but the outcome needs to be realistic. Here are some general guidelines:

- Focus on antioxidant facial treatments with deep hydration. Take care with aggressive peeling agents.
- Recommend daily antioxidant supplementation. See Chapter 10 for more information.
- Medical aesthetic treatments may be more effective, such as dermal fillers, lasers, and daily use of prescription tretinoin.

> If undergoing cosmetic surgery, a client must stop smoking at least one month before the procedure.

ALCOHOL AND THE SKIN

Excessive alcohol intake is detrimental to health and can interfere in a healthy aging program. Daily alcohol intake is recommended at 1 ounce. a day. For example, a 16 ounce beer with a 5% alcohol, introduces approximately 0.08 ounces of alcohol to the system. The liver can burn up to an ounce of alcohol an hour, and levels above this are toxic to the body.[4]

Excessive alcohol use shows up as yellow, dull, dehydrated skin. It does not cause rosacea but does aggravate it. Alcohol also causes vasodilatation, which can increase flushing, and as elasticity weakens telangiectasia can develop. It also depletes the body of essential nutrients and acts as a diuretic, which depletes the body water content.

What to Do for Clients Who Drink

Education is the best approach. Be honest with clients about the improvements that they can see. Improvement of aging symptoms is going to be minimal with a heavy drinker, but hydration and relaxation can be enhanced. Clients know when they have a problem, and it is the esthetician's responsibility to focus on treatment results with information that the client can use at home, not focusing on getting them into treatment. Even if measurable gains cannot be made in the skin while the client is drinking, the effects of facial treatments have the following benefits to the client:

- Relaxation
- Increased lymph movement and microcirculation
- Delivering nutrients to the skin
- Exfoliation
- Hydration

DRUGS AND THE SKIN

Drug usage, both legal and illegal, has profound effects on the skin. There are many resources available on the use of pharmaceuticals and skin reactions, but illegal drug use is rarely discussed. The esthetician may come into contact with clients who are using illegal drugs, and most often there are no immediate reactions within the treatment but occasionally reactions can occur that are unexpected. Rarely do clients admit that they are using illegal drugs; in fact, many do not even disclose the medications that they are using. In this section we will discuss the two most common illegal drugs that may affect the esthetician. Age is not a factor in use; therefore, this section does directly relate to treating aging skin.

Marijuana

Marijuana use is common but still is illegal in the United States with the exception of medical marijuana use in some states. Marijuana is actually the bud and leaves of the Cannabis sativa plant and has been used for thousands of years for medical and spiritual purposes. The United States outlawed marijuana in 1937, but an estimated 14.8 million people in the United States use it. Chances are the esthetician has several clients who are using it.

Marijuana has profound effects on the brain and body. The main chemical component of marijuana is **THC (delta-9-tetrahydrocannabinol)**, which is known to affect the brain's short-term memory, raise anxiety, and affect motor coordination. It is also used to relieve the symptoms of glaucoma, reduce the side effects of cancer treatment, and relieve some symptoms of HIV patients. It has been found to reduce muscle spasms, increase appetite, stop convulsions, and reduce menstrual pain.

No studies have been done on the exact effect of marijuana on the skin, but it can have the same side effects as smoking. As an unregulated substance, there are hundreds of chemicals within marijuana, all with unknown side effects. The effects may be less intense than someone smoking nicotine.

In general, you may see the following within the skin of a marijuana smoker:

- Increased dehydration
- Increased sensitivity
- Increased vasodilatation
- Slow healing response
- Uneven texture and color
- Resistant skin

Generally an esthetician will not know if his or her clients are using marijuana until a reaction happens or repeated treatments do not improve the skin as expected with the clients who have disclosed health information.

When faced with marijuana-smoking clients, the esthetician should act as follows:

- If an esthetician has a trusting relationship with the client, straightforward communication is the best approach. Ask the client if they are using marijuana or other substances.
- Do not judge. An esthetician can decide if he or she still wants to treat the client, but it is not the esthetician's place to preach or otherwise demean the client.
- Explain the side effects of smoking on the skin. Having printed material that outlines the effects of smoking in general to give the client is helpful. Knowledge is power.
- Explain what can be accomplished within treatment parameters. Do not overpromise results even if the client is willing to *do anything*. Without lifestyle changes, improvement is minimal.
- Have the client sign a general liability waiver. This should be a standard practice.

Even if a client is using medical marijuana, choose treatments that support the skin. Focus on hydration and antioxidant therapy to reduce the long-term effects of free radical damage. Stress reduction will be important for these clients as they are usually dealing with a serious chronic condition.

Methamphetamine

Methamphetamine is a powerful stimulant that causes the brain to release a surge of dopamine that can last from six to twenty-four hours. Methamphetamine can come in powder or crystal form and is ingested by inhaling up the nose or smoked. Methamphetamine is also available in pill form, which is less popular.

This illegal drug is an epidemic in the United States, with as many as 1.4 million people using it.[5] The effects on the brain and body are devastating. It is a drug that profoundly affects the skin as well. Chances are that estheticians will not be dealing with someone who is highly addicted to meth; they may be dealing with recreational users or someone recovering from addiction.

Meth is highly addictive and over time destroys **dopamine receptors** in the brain, which will prevent the user from feeling pleasure. This leads to severe depression, and heavy users exhibit extreme paranoia, hyperactivity, aggressiveness, delusions, and hallucinations. Even when a person stops using meth, the damage remains within the brain. Dopamine receptors can grow back, but the cognitive damage remains. Meth destroys tissue and vessels within the body, which leads to distinctive visual signs (Figure 9–7 a and b), such as:

- Tooth decay and loss
- Acne
- Poor healing lesions
- **Excoriations** and sores
- Extreme elastosis and loss of GAGs
- Gaunt and frail appearance; body can look anorexic

dopamine receptors

receptors found in the central nervous sytem and key organs that help regulate dopamine which is essential for proper nerve function. A disruption in dopamine results in mood disorders, poor memory and cognitive dysfunction.

excoriations

a condition in which patients produce skin lesions, scratches, and irritation through repetitive, compulsive picking of their skin.

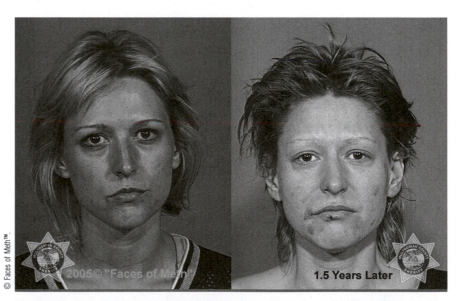

Figure 9–7 The effects of methamphetamine on the brain and body are devastating.

How to Handle Clients on Meth?

Do not perform treatments on heavy meth users. Chances are they will not be seeking self-care services due to their addiction, but if you are faced with a heavy user presenting with the previously listed symptoms, it is best to step away, for the following reasons:

- Personal safety. Meth users exhibit unpredictable behavior.
- Treatments will not work. No improvement can be made on the skin if they are actively using meth.
- Treatments can cause side effects within the body. Meth affects the vascular system profoundly, and many esthetic treatments cause vasodilatation as well as vasoconstriction, which could lead to further damage.

If the client is a recovering addict with extreme visual signs, a combined approach of medical aesthetic procedures such as injectable fillers with esthetic treatments with a focus on exfoliation and hydration can be beneficial.

Lifestyle choices have a profound effect on the body, and the esthetician needs to be aware of what those signs are before performing treatment or creating a healthy aging plan.

▶ ⟩ ⟩ Top Ten Tips to Take to the Clinic

1. Learn the visual symptoms of clients under stress.
2. Keep the treatment room free of clutter and avoid strong smells for a stressed client.
3. Teach your client a quick deep breathing technique.
4. Ask about diet and have information to offer the client.
5. Ask about drug and alcohol use without imposing judgment.
6. Know the signs of smoking in the skin.
7. Know the signs of meth use in the skin.
8. Reduce your own stress levels; clients can see the effects in you as well.
9. Know that many esthetic treatments can help make a negative lifestyle habit less apparent.
10. Do not overpromise results to those that have lifestyle habits that are negative.

Chapter Review Questions

1. Describe stress.
2. What are some of the causes of stress?
3. What is the right amount of sleep?
4. List coping strategies to help manage stress.
5. What are the signs of smoking in the skin?

References

1. Benson, H. (December 5, 1997). "The Relaxation Response: Therapeutic Effect." *Science* 278(5344):1694–5.
2. Cromie, W. (February 2, 2006). "Meditation Is Found to Increase Brain Size." *Harvard Gazette*.
3. Baumann, L. MD., Saghari, S. MD., Weisburg, E. MS. (2009). *Cosmetic Dermatology: Principles and Practice*, 2nd Edition. New York: McGraw Hill Medical.
4. Pugliese, P. MD. (2001). *Physiology of the Skin II*. Carol Stream, IL: Allured Publishing.
5. Suo, S. (October 3, 2004). "Unnecessary epidemic." *The Oregonian*.

Bibliography

Lam, P. (2004). Nutrition: *The Healthy Aging Solution*. Carol Stream, IL: Allured Publishing.

Man-Tu Lee, A., Weiss, D. (2002). *Zen in 10 Simple Lessons*. East Sussex, UK: Barron's Education Services.

Patlak, M. (2005). *Your Guide to Healthy Sleep*. U.S. Department of Health and Human Services. Retrieved from http://www.nhlbi.nih.gov/health/public/sleep/healthy_sleep.pdf.

Websites

www.howstuffworks.com
www.helpguide.org
www.emotional-intelligence.org
www.stress.org

Nutrition for the Skin

Chapter 10

Key Terms

edema

krill

metabolic syndrome

osmotic pressure

Learning Objectives

After completing this chapter, you will be able to:

1. Explain the basics of healthy nutrition.
2. Discuss which supplements and foods to recommend by skin conditions.

metabolic syndrome

three or more disorders related to your metabolism at the same time, which includes obesity (particularly around the waist area having an apple shape), a systolic (top number) blood pressure measurement higher than 120, or a diastolic (bottom number) blood pressure measurement higher than 80, elevated level of triglycerides and low Low Density Lipoprotein, resistance to insulin.

To calculate the number of ounces a client should drink daily, divide the client's body weight by half. For example: 150 lbs/2 = 75 oz of water per day.

■ INTRODUCTION

Healthy nutrition is an essential part of the treatment of aging skin. Many of the symptoms that estheticians see in the skin can be magnified or caused by poor nutrition. Issues of obesity, diabetes, and **metabolic syndrome** affect the skin directly with poor healing, glycation, and reduction in hydration within the skin. A nutritionist should be considered an important professional included in the comprehensive plan presented to the client, but the esthetician can provide basic nutritional information if properly informed.

The basics of a daily healthy diet include (Figure 10–1):

- 50–60 percent carbohydrates
- 15–25 percent healthy fats with less than 10 percent saturated fat
- 15–20 percent protein
- 35–50 grams fiber

It is also important to include adequate water intake, which is generally recommend as 0.5 ounces per pound of body weight. If the client is exercising, in a low ambient humidity environment, smoking, drinking, or taking medications, the amount of water intake should increase.

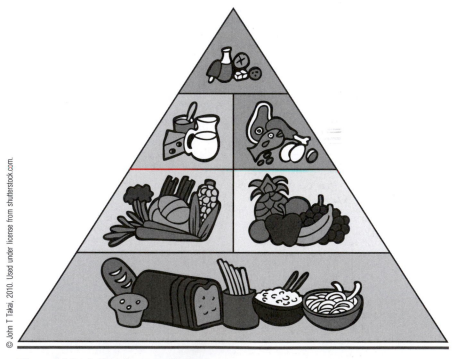

© John T Takai, 2010. Used under license from shutterstock.com.

Figure 10–1 Food pyramid chart.

Depending on the goals of the client, diet modifications can be made to address weight loss, disease prevention, or health improvement. Some general guidelines to follow are:

- **Increase the intake of vegetables and whole grains.** This advice has been given for many years, with many of us groaning as we hear it. The reality is that a vegetarian diet does have substantial health benefits. One does not need to become a vegetarian to gain benefits.
- **Reduce saturated fat intake.** A high-fat diet based on animal protein is also high in saturated fat, which can impact heart health. More insidious is the hydrogenated (trans-fats) fats that are present in many processed foods.
- **Reduce refined sugar.** Obvious sources of sugar are sodas, cakes, and sweets, which should be limited. Look at any processed food, and you will see a tremendous amount of sugar. A good rule to follow is that the sugar content should not be more than the protein content. Avoid sucrose, glucose, maltose, and fructose corn syrup.
- **Reduce sodium and increase potassium intake.** The average diet is high in sodium, which raises blood pressure and can contribute to **edema**. The ratio of sodium to potassium should be 1:2 to maintain constant **osmotic pressure** within the body. Sources of potassium are vegetables and fruit.

When it comes to diet planning, simple physics is still the proven way to approach the challenge:

- To lose weight you must burn more calories than you take in (daily energy input [calories] minus energy spent [exercise, daily activity] equals weight loss)
- To maintain weight, calories in will equal calories expended (daily energy input [calories] equals daily energy expenditure)
- To gain weight, calories in must be more than calories expended (daily energy greater than energy expenditure equals weight gain)

Easy as this system is, it is hard to follow for many millions of people. There is much debate in scientific community about some of the causes of obesity and as many theories about what to eat and when. Here are some simple guidelines that will fit with any diet plan:

Balance: it is important to have balanced nutrition and not focus on one food group. The section on healthy diet guidelines has a balanced approach to follow.

Moderation: portion size is important as well as controlling cravings. To abstain completely from the foods one craves just increases

edema
extracellular water that becomes trapped and causes swelling.

osmotic pressure
hydrostatic pressure caused by a difference in the amounts of solutes between solutions that are separated by a semi-permeable membrane.

desire. Using moderation can help control the intake of those *forbidden* foods. Just adjust calorie intake the next day.

Nutrient density: this means consuming foods with balanced nutrients such as protein, fiber, vitamins, and minerals with lower calorie density. Foods with higher fiber content such as green leafy vegetables (broccoli, cauliflower) and whole grains also help with increasing satiety.

Adequate intake: relates to making sure the basic calorie intake is adequate for daily activity, diet planning goals, and health issues. This includes adequate water intake based on daily activity.

Variety: this keeps the diet interesting and varies the type of nutrients consumed. Consuming the same food all the time leads to boredom and imbalance.

All of these recommendations can be given to the client with a disclaimer to find professional help such as a nutritionist. Each individual has different conditions that need to be taken into account, which are out of scope of practice for the esthetician.

Nutrition Supplements and Recommendations for the Skin

How the skin reacts to diet and hormones is important for the esthetician to understand when designing a healthy aging program for the client. There are more and more nutritional supplements available on the market specific for improving the skin, hair, and nails. Understanding how these products can influence the health of the skin is important when designing a healthy aging program. Supplements can also be another income stream available to the esthetician as well as supporting a client's complete healthy aging lifestyle.

Dietary Supplements That Can Impact Skin
Vitamins

Vitamin A: Regulates growth and differentiation of epithelial cells, inhibits tumor growth, decreases inflammation, and enhances the immune system (Figure 10–2).[1] Beta-carotene is a member of the carotenoid family, which is considered a provitamin. It is the safest and most effective way to get the best vitamin A dosage.

Benefits: Retinol and retinoic acid are applied topically for reversing photoaging, actinic keratosis, pigmentation, and smoothing skin texture. Taken internally, the immune system is enhanced, skin barrier function is improved, and acne is improved. Beta-carotene can provide protection from UV radiation–induced erythema.

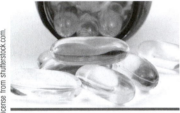

Figure 10–2 Nutritional supplements can be very beneficial to the skin.

© BW Folsom, 2010. Used under license from shutterstock.com.

In 1994 the United States government passed the Dietary Supplement Health and Education Act, which deregulated the marketing of dietary supplements. This has made the manufacturers responsible for maintaining quality and safety. It is important to look for the USP (United States Pharmacopeia) label when picking supplements to use and provide to clients.

Dosage and Cautions: Better to take internally with diet rather than supplementation due to toxicity. A basic multivitamin will enhance the amount needed for health. Do not exceed 10,000 IU. Supplements can cause birth defects if taken during pregnancy. Beta-carotene can be taken in 15–30 mg daily. Good food sources are leafy greens (Figure 10–3), carrots, sweet potatoes, spinach, broccoli, squash, and mangoes.

Biotin: Known as B_7, part of the B vitamin family.

Benefits: Estimated that biotin increases nail thickness up to 25 percent.[2]

Dosage and Cautions: No known cautions; dosage should be 2.5 mg daily.

Niacin: Known as B_3 (nicotinic acid); not created within the body; must be supplied by the diet or supplementation.

Benefits: Essential for the healthy function of the nervous system and skin. Used as treatment for inflammatory diseases and possible treatment for migraines. Causes vasodilatation. Niacinamide is used topically to treat photodamage, inflammation, hyperpigmentation, and dry skin.

Dosage and Cautions: No dosage recommendation beyond the recommended dose of 15–19 mg daily.

D_3: Actually a hormone, activated in the body by sun exposure (Figure 10–4).

Benefits: Helps regulate cellular activity in keratinocytes and immune cells. Increases bone mineral density; prevention of some cancers and a potent antioxidant. Some studies have also shown an improvement in cardiovascular health.

Dosage and Cautions: It is unsafe for vitamin D_3 to be obtained strictly through sun exposure. It takes only a limited amount of time for synthesis to happen; in some areas it is important for supplementation due to lack of year-round sun. The best method is oral capsules (best in gel capsule) in dosages from 600–800 IU daily. Vitamin D levels should be tested by a physician. Foods that can be helpful are fortified milk and milk products, as well as mushrooms.

Antioxidants

Vitamin C: One of the most recognized and studied vitamins, known as ascorbic acid and found in citrus fruits (Figure 10–5).

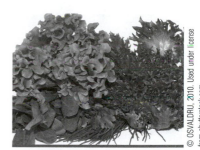

Figure 10–3 Green leafy vegetables are a great source of vitamin A.

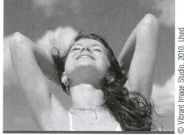

Figure 10–4 Vitamin D_3 is a hormone, activated in the body by sun exposure.

The recent controversy about vitamin D supplementation revolves around calcium supplementation, not D_3 specifically. Clients in climates with little or no sun, who work indoors consistently and have poor immunity should still use supplementation or specific diet strategies to increase this important vitamin.

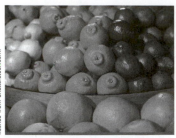

Figure 10–5 Vitamin C, a potent antioxidant, has many benefits to the skin.

Benefits: Potent antioxidant, anti-inflammatory, helps collagen synthesis, helps prevent and treat stretch marks, strengthens immune system, and prevents disease. Topically applied it is photoprotective and essential to an anti-aging program.

Dosage and Cautions: Dosage should be 500 mg two times a day; no known toxicity but stomach side effects if taken in excess.

Vitamin E: Referred to as alpha-tocopherol and is part of the tocopherols and tocotrienols group. Vitamin E naturally occurs in the membranes of cells and organelles and is an important part of sebum.

Benefits: Most significant lipid antioxidant, protects cell membranes from free radical scavengers, helps prevent heart disease, improves skin dryness through skin barrier stabilizing, anti-inflammatory, immune system stimulating, and protection against photodamage.

Dosage and Cautions: There are risks in taking too much. Recommended dose is 400 IU in gel cap form daily. Doses exceeding 3,000 mg can cause bruising. Vitamin E should be discontinued 10 days prior to esthetic medical procedures. This includes injections such as Botox®.[3]

Coenzyme Q10:   Known as ubiquinone, found in all human cells, significant role in creating ATP (adenosine triphosphate), levels decline with age.

Benefits: Assists in energy production, prevents cell death from free radicals by inhibiting lipid peroxidation, suppresses free radical development, slows down the reduction in cellular energy production associated with aging, and reduces wrinkles. Topical CoQ10 reduces wrinkle depth, reduces free radical oxidation, inhibits collagenase in fibroblasts, and is photoprotective.

Dosage and Cautions: Has a stimulatory effect and is recommended to be taken in the morning, 200 mg daily. If taking cholesterol-lowering drug, 400 mg is recommended. Low CoQ10 levels are associated with fatigue and muscle cramping. No toxicity dose identified.[4]

Lycopene: Responsible for the red hue in tomatoes, other red fruits and vegetables, and naturally found in human blood.

Benefits: Antioxidant helps to reduce oxidative damage to tissues. Studies show that it absorbs or slows down the effects of UV radiation and other oxidative stress.[5] It is considered an effective sun protectant when taken internally. It is also known to decrease the risk of cancer and cardiovascular disease.

Dosage and Cautions: Dosage is recommended at 24 mg daily.

Green Tea: A staple in Asian countries, part of the polyphenol group of antioxidants (Figure 10–6). The main compound that gives antioxidant protection is EGCG (epigallocatechin-3-O-gallate).

Benefits: Anti-inflammatory, anticarcinogenic, helps mediate the biochemical pathways that govern cell proliferation, reduces UV-induced immunosuppression and can repair UV-induced DNA damage. Green tea is theorized to help rosacea and pigmentation disorders and prevent irritation from retinoids.

Dosage and Cautions: There is no widely accepted daily supplemental dose, but it is recommended that up to five cups of green tea a day will give significant preventive health benefits. Topical application has been well studied, and it is recommended to use products that have 50–90 percent polyphenol ingredient level, which will make the product dark brown.[6]

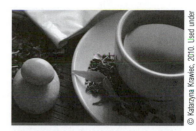

Figure 10–6 Green tea is an antioxidant that is a staple in Asian countries.

Silymarin: Derived from the seeds of the milk thistle plant, part of the polyphenol flavonoid group (Figure 10–7). The main component is silybin and has been used for centuries for medicinal purposes.

Benefits: Antioxidant, anti-inflammatory, anticarcinogenic, and photoprotective. Silymarin is used regularly for liver support. Applied topically it imparts protection against UV-induced skin damage.

Dosage and Cautions: Recommended dose 280–450 mg a day in capsule form or 100–200 mg twice a day if using silymarin-phosphatidylcholine complex, which studies have shown is easier to absorb. Silymarin may interfere with allergy medications, drugs for high cholesterol, anti-anxiety drugs, blood thinners, and some cancer drugs.

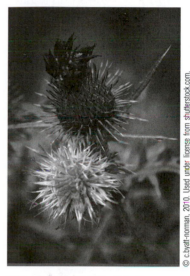

Figure 10–7 Milk thistle applied topically imparts protection against UV-induced skin damage.

Resveratrol: Found in the skin and seed of grapes, berries, peanuts, and red wine and part of the polyphenol phytoalexin group (Figure 10–8). It exists in two forms: trans-resveratrol and cis-resveratrol. Trans-resveratrol is the most stable form.

Benefits: Strong antioxidant, anti-inflammatory, and has potential as a cancer treatment agent. Topical application inhibits free radical damage and is thought to help prevent skin cancer.

Dosage and Cautions: Dosages for humans are currently being studied. A commonly accepted dosage is 20 mg a day. No cautions are reported at this time.

Grape Seed Extract: Part of the polyphenolic flavonoid family or OPC (oligomeric proanthocyanidin complexes), come from the plant

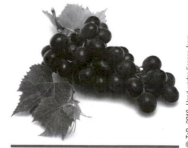

Figure 10–8 Grapes are a strong antioxidant that are also anti-inflammatory and have potential as a cancer treatment agent.

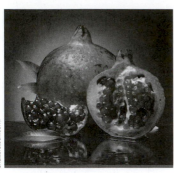

Figure 10–9 Pomegranate extract was one of the first sources of medicine due to its many benefits.

Vitis viniferia or grapes. Grapes have been used for over 6,000 years to treat various medical issues.

Benefits: Antioxidant, anti-inflammatory; used to treat chronic venous insufficiency, edema, high cholesterol, and high blood pressure. Used in cancer prevention. No topical human studies but is thought to reduce UV-induced oxidative stress and is a potent free radical scavenger.

Dosage and Cautions: Daily dosage for the following:

- Free radical protection: 25–150 mg, one to three times daily
- Edema: 200–400 mg for 10–30 days
- Chronic venous insufficiency: 150–300 mg daily

Look for a 95 percent OPC value to make sure supplement is potent. Pregnant or breastfeeding women and clients on blood thinning medications should not take grape seed extract.

Pomegranate Extract: From *Punica granatum*, a fruit native to northern India, Iran, Pakistan, and Afghanistan (Figure 10–9). One of the first sources of medicine and used throughout the world to treat various diseases.

Benefits: Antioxidant, reduces skin inflammation, nourishing and balancing to the skin, and helps rheumatism. Topically applied peel may help dermal rejuvenation; seed oil may help epidermal rejuvenation.

Dosage and Cautions: Eight to twelve ounces of juice daily; if treating disease conditions, 8 oz. of juice. There is no stated dosage for supplements that may be available.

Pycnogenol: Known as pine bark extract, its source is the French maritime pine (Figure 10–10).

Benefits: Antioxidant, anti-inflammatory, anticarcinogenic. It is used topically for skin lightening effects, with oral supplementation improving melasma.

Dosage and Cautions: Dosage should be 25 mg three times a day with meals.

Essential Fatty Acids

These fatty acids are one of the most important supplements needed for good health and have a direct profound impact on the skin.

Omega-3:   These fatty acids are not created in the body and must be supplied with diet and supplementation. They are part of the PUFA (polyunsaturated fatty acids) family and are an essential part of cell

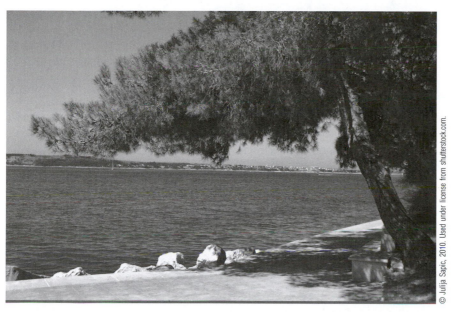

Figure 10–10 Pycnogenol is an antioxidant taken from French maritime pine trees.

krill
common name given to shrimp-like marine crustaceans.

Fish oil supplementation has some environmental aspects that must be considered. Cod is an endangered fish. **Krill** oil is a new supplement that will provide omega-3 benefits without endangering the fish population. It also is known to not cause the unpleasant side effects of fish oil supplements. Flaxseed oil is good too but not a complete source for fatty acid replacement. Alternating between krill and flaxseed as well as fatty fish in the diet is a comprehensive way to get adequate essential fatty acids.

membranes and the skin's barrier. ALA, EPA, and DHA are the primary essential omega-3 fatty acids.

Benefits: Anti-inflammatory, skin hydration, systemic UV radiation protection, and treatment of psoriasis, rosacea, and erythema. Also helps to lower the risks of heart disease, cancer, and arthritis.

Dosage and Cautions: Dosage should be 1,000 mg daily with the supplement having a ration of more EPA versus DHA. Clients on blood thinners should not take omega-3s without doctor supervision. Good food sources are:

- Canola oil
- Fatty fish: albacore tuna, trout, mackerel, menhaden, salmon (Figure 10–11)
- Flaxseed oil/flaxseed
- Hempseed
- Omega-3 eggs
- Seaweed
- Walnuts

Omega-6 Fatty Acids: Examples used to help the skin are borage seed oil and evening primrose oil. These oils are rich in gamma linolenic acid (GLA).

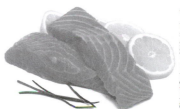

Figure 10–11 Omega-3 fatty acids are not created in the body and must be obtained in the diet or taken as supplements.

Benefits: Soothing of skin inflammation, reduction of dry skin, treatment of eczema, and reduction of irritation.

Dosage and Cautions: Studies have shown skin barrier improvement in doses of 360–720 mg daily for two months.[7]

Minerals and Other Supplements

Zinc: An essential trace mineral found in the body. It must be supplied by diet. Zinc absorption declines with age, gastrointestinal problems.

Benefits: Assists other nutrients in strengthening the skin's barrier function, increases immunity, and helps synthesize retinol binding protein that transmits vitamin A.

Dosage and Cautions: Dosage should be 15 mg for men and 12 mg for women taken daily. Supplements must have a 1:1 ratio of zinc and iron for absorption. Only 20 percent of dietary zinc is absorbed by the body.[8]

Hyaluronic Acid: Abbreviated as HA and also known as hyaluronan, it is the most abundant glycosaminoglycan within the dermis. It can bind water up to 1,000 times its volume and is also found within the joint fluid. Hyaluronic acid is used in injectable fillers as well, and it comes from animal and plant sources.

Benefits: Important for cell growth and membrane receptor function, stabilizes intercellular structures such as collagen and elastin, and helps with joint issues.

Dosage and Cautions: There is no recommended supplementation dosage, and controversy exists about HA taken in supplement form being effective when metabolized through the stomach. It is commonly included in many *joint supplements*, which many clients take. Check labels for source if concerned about consuming animal products.

Glucosamine: Derived from the shells of shellfish, also available as a synthetic derivative *N*-acetylglucosamine. It is important to the production of cartilage and has significant benefits to the skin.

Benefits: Increases skin hydration, reduced wrinkles, enhances wound healing, inhibits tyrosinase production thus helping to reduce hyperpigmentation, and protects the joints.

Dosage and Cautions: Dosage should be 1,500 mg daily with improvements seen in four to six weeks.

DHEA: Dehydroepiandrosterone is a hormone created by the adrenal glands that is used as a precursor to sex hormones. Levels peak around 25 and then decrease with aging. It is used as an anti-aging supplement.

Benefits: Increased sex drive, increased skin hydration, enhances mental clarity, increases metabolism, increases feelings of well-being, and is anti-inflammatory.

Dosage and Cautions: This supplement is a hormone and should be monitored by a physician. Supplementation is not recommended for anyone under 40 years old. Supplements should be taken in the morning to mimic the natural production of DHEA. Men are recommended to take 50 mg daily and women 25 mg daily. Caution should be used with higher dosages.

Making Recommendations

Making recommendations starts with an in-depth consultation. After the concerns of the client are identified, use Table 10–1 chart of foods and supplements for skin types as a quick reference. If clients have medical conditions and are on daily medication, make sure they get clearance from their doctor or pharmacist before taking supplements.

Table 10–1 Chart of foods and supplements by skin condition.

Skin Condition	Goal	Foods to Eat/Avoid	Supplements
Hyperkeratinization	Reduce chronic subclinical inflammation, increase natural lipids in skin.	EFAs (fish oil, fatty fish, flaxseed), seaweed.	Vitamin A, C, E, calcium, zinc, phosphorus, magnesium, iron, zinc. EFAs 1,000–2,000 mg × day, D_3.
Dehydration	Increase cells, ability to retain water, decrease inflammation.	EFAs (fish oil, fatty fish, flaxseed), walnuts, Greek yogurt.	Glucosamine, MSM, hyaluronic acid (joint supplements). EFAs 1,000–2,000 mg × day.
Stage 1 Aging—fine wrinkles, mild elastosis, mild photodamage	Decrease inflammation, increase cells, ability to hold water, increase free radical protection, reduce glycation.	EFAs, (fish oil, fatty fish, flaxseed), green leafy vegetables (spinach), asparagus, celery, eggplant, garlic, onions/leeks, extra virgin olive oil, monounsaturated fat, increase fiber intake. AVOID: simple carbohydrates (sugar), high fat foods, excessive alcohol.	Soy 40 mg 1x, vitamin A, C, E, calcium, zinc, phosphorus, magnesium, iron, zinc. EFAs 1,000–2,000 mg × day, D_3, glucosamine, MSM, hyaluronic acid (joint supplements).

(continued)

Table 10–1 Chart of foods and supplements by skin condition. *(Continued)*

Skin Condition	Goal	Foods to Eat/Avoid	Supplements
Stage 2 Aging—moderate wrinkles, moderate elastosis, early to moderate photodamage	Decrease inflammation, increase cells, ability to hold water, increase natural lipids in skin, increase free radical protection, reduce glycation, support digestive system, balance hormones.	EFAs (fish oil, fatty fish, flaxseed), green leafy vegetables (spinach), asparagus, celery, eggplant, garlic, onions/leeks, extra virgin olive oil, monounsaturated fat, increase fiber intake. AVOID: simple carbohydrates (sugar), high fat foods, excessive alcohol, processed foods.	Soy 40 mg 1x, vitamin A, C, E, calcium, zinc, phosphorus, magnesium, iron, zinc. EFAs 1,000–2,000 mg × day, D_3, glucosamine, MSM, hyaluronic acid (joint supplements), probiotic supplements, DHEA.
Stage 3 Aging—moderate to deep wrinkles, severe elastosis, severe photodamage	Decrease inflammation, increase cells, ability to hold water, increase natural lipids in skin, increase free radical protection, reduce glycation, support digestive system, balance hormones, support liver function.	EFAs, lycopene (tomatoes), lutein (spinach, kale, broccoli), extra virgin olive oil, increase fiber intake, fatty fish. AVOID: simple carbohydrates (sugar), high fat foods, excessive alcohol, processed foods.	Soy 40 mg 1x, vitamin A, C, E, calcium, zinc, phosphorus, magnesium, iron, zinc. EFAs 1,000–2,000 mg × day, D_3, glucosamine, MSM, hyaluronic acid (joint supplements), probiotic supplements, DHEA, silymarin.
Hyperpigmentation	Reduce inflammation, increase free radical protection.	Ellagic acid (pomegranate).	Grape seed extract, Pycnogenol 25 mg 3x.
Rosacea	Reduce chronic inflammation, support digestive system.	Increase fiber intake, Greek yogurt, kefir. AVOID: spicy food, alcohol, simple carbohydrates (sugar), processed foods.	D_3, EFAs, B vitamins, probiotic supplements.
Acne	Balance hormones, reduce inflammation, and support digestive system.	PUFAs (fish oil, green leafy vegs), beta carotene—vitamin A (carrots, spinach, sweet potatoes, mangos), soybeans. AVOID: iodine, milk, simple carbohydrates (sugar).	D_3, Antioxidants—A, C, E, probiotic supplements. AVOID: iodine supplements, DHEA.

> > > **Top Ten Tips to Take to the Clinic**

1. Healthy nutrition is an important part of treating aging skin.

2. Diets low in refined sugar will improve aging skin.

3. Diets high in complex carbohydrates are essential for aging skin.

4. Increase monounsaturated fat intake and reduce saturated fat intake for healthy skin.

5. Reduce sodium intake and increase potassium to aid in healthy skin as this will also reduce edema.

6. Clients on a vegetarian diet are prone to have essential fatty acid deficiency which will show as hyperkeratinized or dehydrated skin.

7. Dietary supplements are necessary for healthy skin and to slow aging.

8. Dose, consistency of use, and quality will determine whether the supplementation program works.

9. When supplementing for treating aging skin, allow six months to see improvement.

10. Antioxidants in food as well as supplement form are essential.

Chapter Review Questions

1. What are the best supplement recommendations for aging skin?
2. What is the recommended water intake?
3. What foods and drinks should clients with rosacea skin avoid?
4. What foods should skin prone to acne avoid?
5. What do dietary recommendations always start with?

References

1. Baumann, L. MD., Saghari, S. MD., Weisburg, E. MS. (2009). *Cosmetic Dermatology: Principles and Practice*, 2nd Edition. New York: McGraw Hill Medical.
2. Baumann, L. MD., Saghari, S. MD., Weisburg, E. MS. (2009). *Cosmetic Dermatology: Principles and Practice*, 2nd Edition. New York: McGraw Hill Medical.
3. Baumann, L. MD., Saghari, S. MD., Weisburg, E. MS. (2009). *Cosmetic Dermatology: Principles and Practice*, 2nd Edition. New York: McGraw Hill Medical.
4. Baumann, L. MD., Saghari, S. MD., Weisburg, E. MS. (2009). *Cosmetic Dermatology: Principles and Practice*, 2nd Edition. New York: McGraw Hill Medical.
5. Baumann, L. MD., Saghari, S. MD., Weisburg, E. MS. (2009). *Cosmetic Dermatology: Principles and Practice*, 2nd Edition. New York: McGraw Hill Medical.

6. Baumann, L. MD., Saghari, S. MD., Weisburg, E. MS. (2009). *Cosmetic Dermatology: Principles and Practice*, 2nd Edition. New York: McGraw Hill Medical.

7. Baumann, L. MD., Saghari, S. MD., Weisburg, E. MS. (2009). *Cosmetic Dermatology: Principles and Practice*, 2nd Edition. New York: McGraw Hill Medical.

8. Baumann, L. MD., Saghari, S. MD., Weisburg, E. MS. (2009). *Cosmetic Dermatology: Principles and Practice*, 2nd Edition. New York: McGraw Hill Medical.

Bibliography

Corbin, C., Welk, G., Corbin, W., Welk, K. (2006). *Fundamental Concepts of Fitness and Wellness*, 2nd Edition. New York: McGraw Hill Publishers.

Lam, P. (2004). *Nutrition: The Healthy Aging Solution*. Carol Stream, IL: Allured Publishing.

Thornfeldt, C. MD., Bourne, K. LE. (2010). *The New Ideal in Skin Health: Separating Fact from Fiction*. Carol Stream, IL: Allured Publishing.

Websites

www.umm.edu
www.webmd.com
www.lef.org

Fitness—The True Healthy Aging Cure

Chapter 11

Key Terms

human growth
  hormone (hGH)
rate of perceived
  exertion (RPE)

yoga
Swami Sivananda
  Rhada
Pilates

Tai chi (Tai Chi
  Chuan)
Tan Tein

Learning Objectives

After completing this chapter, you will be able to:

1. Understand how exercise affects the skin.
2. Learn the basic principles of exercise.
3. Identify the types of exercise that provide benefits to the skin.

▪ THE BENEFITS OF FITNESS

We are constantly being urged by experts in the wellness community to exercise on a daily basis. The reasons vary from weight loss to improving general health. One benefit often overlooked is its positive effects on aging skin. There is no doubt that exercise is important, what is hard to understand is what type is more effective and why. There are so many common myths and different approaches to fitness it is easy for your client to give up trying to get physically fit. It is helpful for the esthetician to be educated about the importance of fitness in order to direct clients to the appropriate expert and stress the benefits for their appearance as well physical health. The following information will give the esthetician general information about physical fitness guidelines and a description of some of the most common exercise types.

▪ HOW EXERCISE AFFECTS THE SKIN

One of the main benefits of exercise on the skin is the increase of circulation to both the lymphatic as well as vascular system. The circulatory system is the main way that nutrients reach the cells. The lymph system is important not only to the immune system but also for moving fluid to hydrate the cells. When the cells are not fully nourished and hydrated the skin's barrier and cellular regeneration is impacted in a negative manner. This leads to dehydration, thinning skin density, and muscle atrophy, which can trigger loss of elasticity, wrinkles, and vascular issues.

Another benefit of exercise on the skin is the reduction of stress. The stress reaction with in the body is very detrimental when uncontrolled. Long-term chronic stress wreaks havoc not only mentally but physically as well. In 2004 a study was done proving the correlation between chronic stress and premature aging (Figure 11–1). It was found that chronic stress raises the level of oxidative stress within the body and shortens telomeres. Healthy women who reported low levels of stress had longer telomeres, while women who reported chronic stress had shorter telomeres equivalent to a decade in aging.[1]

Chronic stress also leads to subclinical inflammation, which is also implicated in premature aging and disease. Refer to the inflammation theory of aging in Chapter 4. Stress can also cause depression and

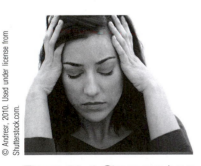

Figure 11–1 Stress can have a very detrimental effect on our skin and body.

anxiety, which can be temporary or turn into a chronic disorder. Exercise will help the body maintain homeostasis when confront from multiple stressors and should be considered an important part of any healthy aging program.

Exercise can also increase the secretion of **human growth hormone (hGH),** which begins to decrease as we age. hGH is involved with most physiological processes within the body and has an impact on fat metabolism, muscle mass, bone density, and collagen formation and maintenance. hGH is secreted in several pulses throughout the day, with sleep and exercise known as the most natural ways to boost its production. Scientists are still unsure how hGH is stimulated by exercise and there are many ongoing studies into this important hormone. One of the current recommendations is to exercise vigorously for at least 10 minutes during a normal workout session. Serious athletes will train multiple times throughout the day with bursts of high intensity in order to increase hGH secretion. There are supplements and diet changes that are known to influence the secretion of hGH. See Chapter 10 for more information on nutrition.

human growth hormone (hGH)

hGH is a hormone involved with most physiological processes within the body and has an impact on fat metabolism, muscle mass, bone density, and collagen formation and maintenance.

What Works?

A balanced approach to fitness is the one that seems to be the most effective for maintaining consistent long-term results. A balanced approach consists of cardiovascular, strength training, and stretching. Strength training is especially important for menopausal women as building muscle will also help strengthen bones, which will reduce the chance of getting osteoporosis. It also helps to raise the basal metabolic rate, which tends to decline as we get older. This can help with maintaining a healthy weight and reduce obesity.

The type of exercise is dependent on the client and what his or her personal physical health can handle. The U.S. Department of Health and Human Services recommends the following guidelines for fitness:

Healthy Adults
Beginners:
150 minutes (2 hours and 30 minutes) moderate intensity aerobic activity or 75 minutes (1 hour and 15 minutes) of vigorous intensity aerobic activity. Performed in at least 10-ten minute increments weekly and can be combined intensities.

RPE	How It Feels		Intensity Level
1	Rest		Light intensity
2	Very light		Light intensity
3	Light		Moderate
4	Fairly light		Moderate intensity
5	Somewhat hard	Speaking or singing is challenging	Moderate intensity
6	Somewhat hard		Vigorous intensity
7	Hard		Vigorous intensity
8	Extremely hard	Cannot speak without difficulty	Vigorous intensity
9	Very hard		Vigorous intensity
10	Maximal exertion		Vigorous intensity

© Milady, a part of Cengage Learning.

Figure 11–2 U.S. Department of Health and Human Services recommended guidelines for fitness.

Advanced:

300 minutes (5 hours) moderate intensity aerobic activity or 150 minutes (2 hours and 30 minutes) of vigorous intensity aerobic activity.

In addition, strength training should be included of a moderate to high intensity two or more days per week.

The easiest way to determine workout intensity is the **rate of perceived exertion** or RPE. RPE is based on how the client feels during exercise and rates the intensity on a scale of 1–10. Figure 11–2 represents guidelines on determining workout intensity.

In order for a fitness program to be successful it is important to include activities that a client enjoys and will not cause injury. The focus should be on building an active lifestyle that will accumulate at 30 minutes of moderate physical activity. For example, vacuuming for one hour with a body weight of 180 pounds will burn 205 calories. The daily goal for physical fitness is 150–300 calories. This of course would be considered a light to moderate activity, so adding a short burst of intense or vigorous activity such as using an elliptical trainer for 20 minutes at 2–3 rpms minimum will be very effective. See Figure 11–3 for a list of common activities and their calorie-burning potential. Working out in group situations (Figure 11–4) also seems to be very helpful for some people, as well as outdoor activity when the weather permits.

rate of perceived exertion (RPE)

a system of determining workout intensity based on how the client feels during exercise and rates the intensity on a scale of 1-10.

Daily Activity	Calories Burned
Shopping with cart	1 hr = 243 kcal
Brushing teeth	2 min = 5.2 kcal
Dusting house	30 min = 80 kcal
Folding clothes	30 min = 72 kcal
Mopping floor	30 min = 153 kcal
Vacuuming	20 min = 56 kcal
Mowing the lawn	1 hr = 324 kcal

© Milady, a part of Cengage Learning.

Figure 11–3 Chart of calorie-burning lifestyle activities.

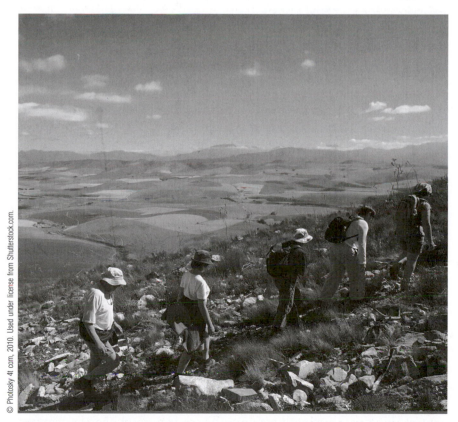

© Photosky 4t com, 2010. Used under license from Shutterstock.com.

Figure 11–4 Working out in group situations can be very helpful for some people.

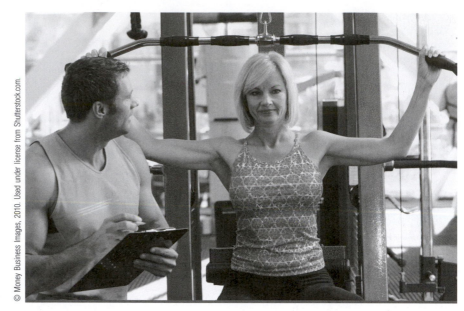

© Money Business Images, 2010. Used under license from Shutterstock.com.

Figure 11–5 Personal trainers can be very helpful in supporting exercising goals.

Personal Trainers

Another approach that may work well is hiring a personal trainer. Personal trainers can be an asset to an esthetician's team of anti-aging experts and a valuable source for referrals. Most trainers can be found at the local gym, while some have independent businesses (Figure 11–5). They usually work on an hourly basis but can have long-term packages available, too. Some states require personal trainers to be licensed, others do not. Make sure you check with your state licensing board for the details. A personal trainer should have a certification.

Strength Training

Strength training is the use of free weights, resistance bands, or weight machines to build muscle density, strength, and endurance. Strength training should be performed at least two days a week, with optimal benefits obtained by working up to four days a week. There are many programs available, from using free weights to resistance bands. The goal in the beginning is to focus on body form during each exercise in order to achieve a safe, injury-free workout. It would be beneficial to suggest to a client that they use a professional personal trainer when first working with strength training. There is a good chance of injury if the exercises are not performed correctly.

Guidelines

Most benefits can be accomplished by performing 8–12 repetitions for each major muscle group; 1–6 reps with heavy weight will build muscle strength, 8–12 reps with moderate weight will increase muscle size, and 15–20 reps with light weight will build muscular endurance. The exercises are completed in sets. A set is a group of repetitions and are completed in groups of 3 different exercise movements or in what are called supersets. This is a group of exercises per area of the body repeated without rest. It is important to work the larger muscle groups first, such as legs before moving on to smaller muscles such as biceps (Figure 11–6). This limits the chance of injury from fatigue.

Recovery time is as important as correct form. Muscles grow during the recovery time and if they are overworked it can create a catabolic effect on the muscle that causes weakening of the muscle. Recovery time is usually 48 hours and can be longer in those will injuries or conditions such as fibromyalgia. Due to the recovery time needed, most strength training programs will split up body parts. There are programs that will allow a beginner to work the entire body with basic weight training exercises. These programs are designed for those that have limited time. Figure 11–7 demonstrates an example of a typical whole body strength training program.

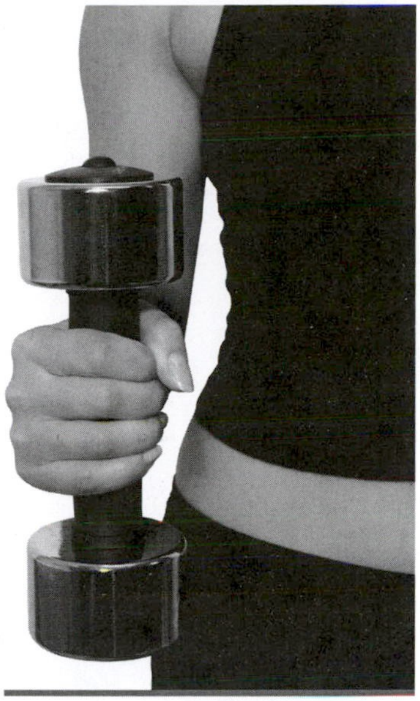

Figure 11–6 Strength training builds muscle density, strength, and endurance.

Full body weight training program		
Area worked	**Exercise**	**Sets/reps**
Core	Swiss ball crunch	3/12
Glutes/hamstrings—curling movements	Barbell deadlift	3/12
Upper back—pulling movements	Barbell row	3/12
Quads—up & down movements	Squats	3/12
Chest—pressing up movements	Barbell bench press	3/12
Lats—pulling movements	Lat pulldown	3/12
Arms—pulling and pressing down movements	Bicep curl, tricep pressdown	3/12
Shoulders—pressing up movements	Shoulder press	3/12

Remember to rest one minute between sets and have at least 24/48 hours of recovery time.

Figure 11–7 A beginner's strength training routine.

Benefits:

The benefits from strength training are varied and can affect each person differently. In general the benefits include:

- Increased metabolic rate. Muscle requires more calories to function.
- Decreased risk of osteoporosis, heart disease, and diabetes.
- Improved posture.
- Increased strength and endurance.
- Slows down the muscle loss that happens as you age.
- Relieves stress.
- Reduces fatigue.
- Improves self-image and self-esteem.
- Increases mental focus.
- Better looking skin.
- Reduction in the appearance of cellulite.

Yoga

yoga
an ancient system of spiritual practice that includes body strengthening, which started as early as 3000 B.C.

Swami Sivananda Radha
yoga guru who modified the five principles of yoga for western culture.

Yoga is an ancient system of spiritual practice which includes body strengthening that started as early as 3000 B.C. In Western society yoga has become a mainstream fitness program without any spiritual or religious connection. There are many yoga paths to follow, from the Western form taken from hatha yoga to truly spiritual practices such as kundalini yoga. The focus is to unite body and mind and create a sense of peace within. Practice can be done at home or in a class, daily or several times a week (Figure 11–8). The fitness level of the individual will determine the type of program to do, but everyone and any fitness level can do yoga.

Guidelines

If yoga is a new physical fitness routine, going to a class to start will help the client learn the fundamentals of yoga and proper form needed to be successful.

There are five principles of yoga that have been modified for Western culture. The following principles were created by yoga guru **Swami Sivananda Radha** in the 1970s:

- **Savasana**—proper relaxation.
- **Asanas**—proper physical fitness.
- **Pranayama**—proper breathing.

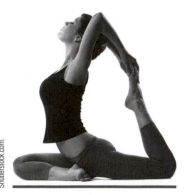

Figure 11–8 Yoga focuses to unite body and mind for an increased sense of peace.

- **Proper diet**—many focus on a non-animal diet and food as medicine.
- **Dhyana**—positive thinking and meditation.

Yoga can be performed on a daily basis and results can be seen in as little as three days a week of consistant practice. There are many different styles and types of yoga and instruction is important when first starting a routine. The following exercise depicts a quick 10-minute beginning program designed by esthetician and yoga instructor Renee Harvey.

BEGINNER'S YOGA ROUTINE (10 MINUTES)

Check with your healthcare provider to make sure any new form of exercise is appropriate for you. Yoga is always done at the level you are comfortable, it should never cause pain. All poses, or asanas, can be modified with or without props so that they are safe with proper alignment. A yoga mat will help prevent slipping for standing poses. You may wish to use extra padding under the knees or ankles. Yoga helps develop strength and flexibility over time.

1. Begin comfortably seated, either cross-legged on the floor (a folded blanket may be placed under hips so that knees are at a lower level than the hips). Place your hands palms up or down on your knees.

    Alternatively, you may sit comfortably in a chair with your feet flat on the floor.

2. Start to become aware of your breathing, notice the coolness of the air as you inhale and the warmth of the air as you slowly exhale.

3. Continue to breathe with awareness. As you breathe begin to release expectations about this yoga session. Focus on your breathing, soften your face, your eyes, and release your shoulders away from your ears.

4. Slowly as you exhale, gently tuck your chin onto your chest; hold this position for three breaths. After three breaths, inhale and slowly bring your head back to center. Exhale, release your head slowly to the right, and become aware of any sensation in the neck muscles as you exhale. After three breaths, inhale your head back to center. Notice, without judgment, any area of tension. Exhale; release your head to the left for three relaxed

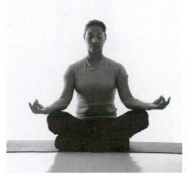

A beginner's yoga program

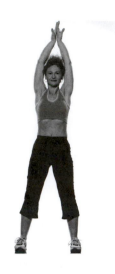

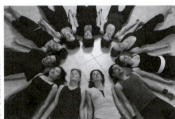

breaths. Inhale your head back to center. Inhale; gently tilt your face upward, exhale back to center.

5. Gently with your hands, raise your knees, feet flat on the floor. Softly cup your hands around the sides of your knees and gently exhale, gently round spine, bringing head toward knees, as you inhale, slowly straighten and lengthen spine as you release the chest muscles. Repeat three times, slowly.

6. Slowly straighten your legs in front of you for seated forward bend, or paschimottanasana. Sit bones are firmly on the floor, sitting tall, and shoulders relaxed. Inhale your arms up and hinge forward from the hips, keeping the spine neutral and head remaining aligned with the spine. Your knees may be slightly bent. With each inhale lengthen the spine, with each exhale allow the torso to release toward the knees. After three breath cycles, inhale and slowly return to neutral position.

7. Slowly make your way to standing position, feet hips-width apart in mountain pose (tadasana). Your knees are soft, pelvis in neutral position, arms at your sides, palms facing forward, shoulders away from ears. Rock back and forth on your feet, exploring their connection to the earth as they stabilize your body. You are standing soft and strong at the same time.

8. Inhale your arms straight out in front of you and above your head in the air, lengthening through fingertips; shoulders remain relaxed, away from ears. Exhale; hinging forward from the hips, fold forward. You may use support blocks and/or knees may be slightly bent. Each inhale, notice the spine lengthening from fingertips through spine and spine through backs of the legs to the feet. Each exhalation, allow your torso to release closer to your thighs.

9. Inhale, reach up through fingertips to flat back (back is parallel to the floor), exhale, fold back down as before.

10. Bend your knees, slowly roll up to standing position, one vertebrae at a time, inhale your arms up, release down into prayer position.

11. Make your way back to the floor; lie quietly for a few moments in corpse pose (savasana). You may cover yourself with a blanket to stay warm.

12. Turn onto your right side, rest for a few moments, and when you are ready, slowly make your way to a seated position. Sit quietly for a few moments.

Benefits:

- Toned, flexible body.
- Increased lymphatic and blood flow.
- Increased muscle tone.
- Reduction of the appearance of cellulite.
- Reduced stress.
- Increased energy.
- Reduction of pain through an increase in endorphin secretion.
- Promotes a healthy glandular system.

Pilates

Pilates is a form of exercise developed by Joseph Pilates during World War I. Joseph was held in an interment camp in England during the war and developed floor exercises using common items to maintain his health as well as help others with injuries. The focus of Pilates is to develop a strong core strength utilizing the six Pilates principles (Figure 11–9). The core is the internal muscles of the abdomen and the back. When the core is strong the body will be more stable and back pain can be reduced if not eliminated.

Pilates
form of exercise created by Joseph Pilates which focuses on core strength.

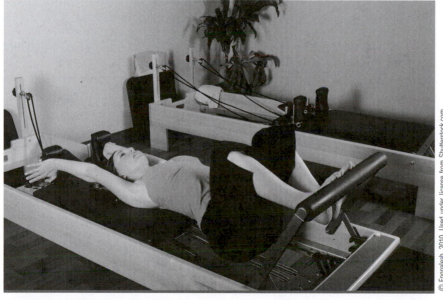

© Eponaleah, 2010. Used under license from Shutterstock.com.

Figure 11–9 Pilates focuses on developing strong core strength in the abdominal and back muscles.

Guidelines:

The six Pilates principles are what separate Pilates from many other exercise programs. The six principles are:

1. **Centering**: this refers to bringing the focus to the center or core of the body. This area is usually described as the area between the navel and pubic bone.
2. **Control**: control relates to muscles used during the exercise. Each movement requires complete muscular control in all range of motion.
3. **Concentration**: incorporates mind techniques that require focus on the present. Each movement requires concentration for maximum benefits.
4. **Breath**: Pilates requires full belly breaths with each movement. It has been described as using the lungs as bellows, forcing the air in and out with strength.
5. **Precision**: throughout each exercise a precise body form is sustained throughout each movement. This helps with getting maximum benefit from each movement, not relying on multiple repetitions for a benefit.
6. **Flow**: Pilates is performed with fluid and grace much like a dance. Flow is important to get maximum benefit from Pilates and connects all of the principles together. If you are not practicing correct form, for example, your movements will not flow together. Flow also refers to energy "flowing" to all parts of the body.

Pilates can be performed on a daily basis with each program being modified. For example, if a high-intensity Pilates program is performed, the next day the routine can be modified to a lighter, slower flowing routine. There are daily 10-minute routines that make this easier as well. Most people will start out with 3–4 days a week, which is still very effective if the six principles are adhered to.

Benefits:

- Develops core strength.
- Increases flexibility.
- Helps reduce back pain through strengthening core, spine alignment, and increased endorphin release.
- Improves posture.
- Reduces stress.
- Increases body awareness.
- Creates strength by bulking up muscle.
- Increases energy.
- Promotes weight loss.

Tai Chi

Tai Chi, also known as **Tai Chi Chuan**, is an ancient martial arts form that is used as a gentle meditative exercise. There are many different styles and over 100 types of movements, all are done in a gentle rhythmic flow with focused deep breathing. The goal is to create an inner sense of calm and focus only on the present moment. It is like a "moving meditation," which is very valuable at controlling stress. Tai Chi also develops fine motor control, which has a tendency to weaken as we age, and helps to strengthen balance. The styles that focus on martial arts are faster paced and very in depth. Training to master these styles can take a lifetime. When studied as a martial art, the focus is not explosive offense when attacking but a soft approach, often using the opponent's own momentum to diffuse the attack.

Asian culture believes that we have an energy called chi that circulates within our body through meridians. The energy is stored in the lower abdomen, called "**Tan Tien.**" They believe that when we are younger we have a healthy abundant amount of chi but as we get older the meridians become blocked and chi is reduced. This leads to ill health and disease. Tai Chi is used to increase the flow of chi and help the body reduce blockages. Tai Chi is also based on the Yin/Yang balance of energy. Yin is the female or soft side while Yang represents the male or hard side. As the flow of energy is balanced so is Yin and Yang.

Guidelines

Initial training starts with the slow and flowing movements of the Tai Chi style chosen. Advanced study combines both the hard and fast movements for self-defense. The most popular style is the Yang style.

There is no special equipment to use and attire is loose flowing and comfortable. Tai Chi can be performed anywhere and some simplified routines do not require a large space. Tai Chi can be performed daily, with benefits reported in as little as two 60-minute sessions a week.

Posture is very important in the practice of Tai Chi. Posture guidelines are:

- Whole body relaxed with head held high.
- Shoulders should be relaxed but not forced back.
- Pelvis should be slightly tilted forward, bottom tucked under for a straight spine.
- Center of gravity should be focused on your core, with back straight.
- One foot should not be moved while shifting weight to the other foot.

Tai Chi
also referred to as *Tai Chi Chuan*; an ancient martial arts form that is used as a gentle meditative exercise.

Tan Tien
chi energy stored in the lower abdomen.

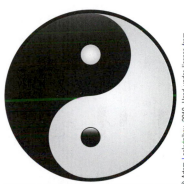

© Artem Loskutnikov, 2010. Used under license from Shutterstock.com.

Figure 11–10 Yin/Yang symbol represents the balance of male and female energies or chi.

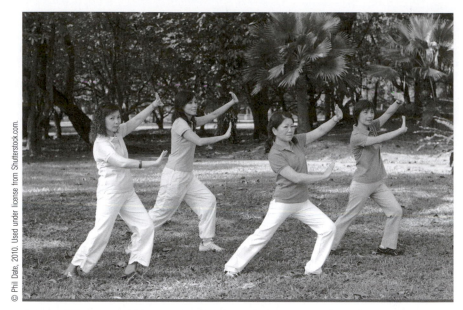

Figure 11–11 Tai Chi class.

- Breathing should be slow and deep, belly breathing as used in yoga.
- In breath is used with open movements, with exhale used in pushing or closing movements.

There are many videos, books, and classes available for details on a working routine. The best resource is a local class or DVD; it is easier to learn by watching this particular exercise form.

Benefits:

- Reduction of pain from osteoarthritis: There is scientific evidence to support that Tai Chi can reduce pain in the knee from osteoarthritis. Chenchen Wang et al.[2] used one-hour Yang-Style Tai Chi practice two times a week to see a significant reduction in pain, and improvement in depression and physical functioning.
- Stress reduction: Tai Chi is considered a moving meditation and will help focus the mind in the present moment.
- Increased energy (chi).
- Improved concentration.
- Improved sleep.
- Increased flexibility.
- Improved heart and lung function.
- Strengthened bones, muscles, and joints.

Cardiovascular Training

Cardiovascular training is also known as aerobic training and is thought to be the most important form of physical fitness training. Cardiovascular training affects all body systems, such as the cardiovascular system (heart), vascular system (blood flow and lymph), respiratory system (lungs), and muscular system (muscles). Cardiovascular training can encompass such activities as running, aerobic dance, cycling, walking, swimming, and equipment work on the elliptical trainer, treadmill, and recumbent bike.

Guidelines

Cardiovascular training should be done three to six days per week at between 55–90% of your maximum heart rate for 20–60 minutes. The formula for determining maximum heart rate is maxHR = 208 − (0.7 × age). To determine 55–90% range, use the following formula: maxHR × % = bpm.[3] See Figure 11–12 for an example.

Another way to determine the intensity of a workout is the rate of perceived exertion, also referred to as workout intensity.

Benefits:

- Increased endurance.
- Strengthened heart muscle.
- Strengthened respiratory system.
- Increased lymphatic circulation.
- Increased muscle strength.
- Stress reduction.
- Increased circulation.
- Weight loss.
- Decreased depression and anxiety.
- Prevention of heart disease, diabetes, and high blood pressure.
- Increased secretion of endorphins. This increases a feeling of well-being and reduces pain.

> Cardiovascular training is one of the fastest ways to improve the skin. The increased blood and lymph flow help hydrate the skin as well as speed up cellular processes.

Formula	Example
maxHR = 208 − (0.7 × age) To determine 55–90% range, use the following formula: maxHR × % = bpm	(0.7 × 41) = 28.7 41 yr old 208−28.7 = 179.3 maxHR Exercise should be within the 55–85% range 179.3 × 85% = 152 bpm Above this oxygen is depleted

© Milady, a part of Cengage Learning.

Figure 11–12 The formula for determining maximum heart rate.

Case Study

The case study from the previous chapters gave some key clues to the client's lifestyle:

- Travels a lot
- Under stress

The client's concerns are primarily related to aging. Based on this subjective information from our client, and the knowledge of the basic fitness options available, the recommendation would be:

☐ Yoga—stress reduction, strength, flexibility (skin will improve with decreased cortisol and improved microcirculation)

☐ Pilates (can be done in a hotel room with no equipment)—builds muscle strength

☐ Cardiovascular training—increased oxygen intake, stress reduction, increased blood flow (skin will improve with increased microcirculation, fibroblasts will be stimulated by hGH)

The esthetician would then refer the client to a fitness expert or let the client do her own research. This completes a healthy aging consultation!

When advising a client to increase physical exercise, make sure that they get permission from their doctor when they present with any of the following in their health history:

Heart disease

Obesity

Diabetes

Injury

High blood pressure

Cancer

An esthetician is not required to provide the client with a detailed fitness routine, only know the basic information to educate the client. Since skin is our focus, knowing how fitness affects the skin is very important. To maximize any healthy aging program it must be included.

▶ ▷ ▷ Top Ten Tips to Take to the Clinic

1. A fitness program is essential for aging skin.
2. Weight training should be performed two to four days a week.
3. Yoga will reduce stress and improve skin.
4. Pilates improves core strength and can reduce back pain.
5. Tai Chi is a moving meditation that can reduce arthritis pain.
6. Cardiovascular training improves skin quickly.
7. Always look at the client's lifestyle when recommending type of exercise.
8. Recommend clients to consult a physician before starting an exercise program if health issues have been identified.
9. Have a fitness expert that is part of your team of experts to refer to.
10. A balanced approach to fitness is the best plan to have.

Chapter Review Questions

1. What benefits does exercise provide skin?

2. How many days per week should strength training be done?

3. What is the recommended plan for beginner physical fitness described by the government?

4. How many days per week can yoga be done?

5. What is hGH?

6. Why is hGH important to skin?

7. Why is chronic stress bad for the body?

References

1. Epel, et al. (December 7, 2004). "Accelerated Telomere Shortening in Response to Life Stress." *PNAS Psychology* Vol. 101, no. 49.

2. Wang, Chenchen, et al. (2008). "Tai Chi Exercise Is Effective in Treating Knee Osteoarthritis: A Randomized Controlled Trial." *Osteoarthritis and Cartilage* 16: s32–s33.

3. Corbin, C., Welk, G., Corbin, W., Welk, K. (2006). *Fundamental Concepts of Fitness and Wellness*, 2nd Edition. New York: McGraw Hill Publishers.

Bibliography

Bryant, G., James, L. (2006). *Simply Tai Chi.* Heatherton, Victoria, Australia: Hinkler Books.

Khalsa, S. K. (2001). *KISS: Guide to Yoga.* New York: DK Publishing.

Andes, K. (1995). *A Woman's Book of Strength: An Empowering Guide to Total Mind/Body Fitness.* New York: The Berkley Publishing Group.

Linguvic, W. (2005). *Lean, Long, and Strong: The 6-Week Strength-Training, Fat-Burning Program for Women.* New York: Holtzbrinck Publisher.

Websites

www.hhs.gov

www.webmd.com

www.about.com

The Green Approach
to Healthy Aging

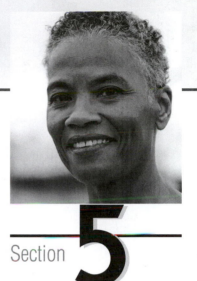

Section **5**

Organic Skin Care

Key Terms

Ecocert
green chemistry
National Organic
  Program (NOP)
organic

Organic and
  Sustainable
  Industry
  Standards
  (OASIS)

stoichiometric

Learning Objectives

After completing this chapter, you will be able to:

1. Discuss whether or not organic products are effective at treating aging skin.

2. Discuss the basics about what is considered organic.

3. Outline the guidelines for certification.

▪ ORGANIC PRODUCTS

Organic is the new marketing buzzword that has created interest and confusion, especially in relation to skin care. Clients request organic products but most people really have no idea what the term entails. Although an organic lifestyle is healthy and has many health benefits, it is hard to translate those standards to the personal care market, including professional-level products. There are a few manufacturers who have mastered this marketing approach but results can be elusive to quantify.

A healthy holistic approach to skin care and overall daily living is an approach that deserves study and reflection. It can be an important part of a healthy aging program and facts and information are needed to wade through the marketing and hype that accompany much of the anti-aging market.

The Meaning of the Term Organic

The term *organic* describes a class of chemicals with a carbon basis (once a living organism). *Organic* as a marketing term is different. When it comes to food labeling the requirements are strict, and the U.S. Department of Agriculture (USDA) imposes fines when they discover a company making claims that are false. There are no USDA guidelines for claiming that a cosmetic product is organic, but manufacturers make that claim when using USDA-certified organic agricultural ingredients. Manufacturers can use any seal that they choose that could indicate organic and natural, as there are no legal guidelines that govern such claims. See Figures 12–1 and 12–2 for examples of a 100 percent natural seal and a certified organic seal.

Does Organic Skin Care Work on Aging Skin?

Can organic products affect mature skin? That answer is not simple. It depends on the issue that the client is dealing with. If you understand the physiology of the skin, then determining whether or not the product will work will be easier. This refers back to Chapter 5 and the structure and function of each layer of the skin. Based on that information, the importance of the acid mantle and stratum corneum cannot be overlooked when treating an aging skin. With an impaired acid mantle, the skin will not be able to maintain hydration within the epidermis, which in turn has a cascade effect on multiple biological processes including enzymatic reactions and inflammation. This process has a

Organic
used to describe a class of chemicals with a carbon basis, or living organism.

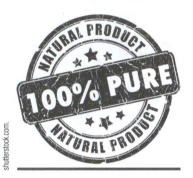

© Arcady, 2010. Used under license from shutterstock.com.

Figure 12–1 Manufacturers can choose any 100% natural seal as there are no legal guidelines that govern such claims.

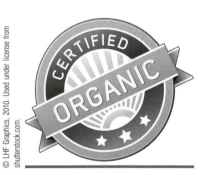

© LHF Graphics, 2010. Used under license from shutterstock.com.

Figure 12–2 Certified organic seals are often used when manufacturers claim the organic ingredients used make a cosmetic product organic.

detrimental effect on aging skin and is the first place that an esthetician should start to improve aging skin.

With that in mind, it is important to look at the four key points of cosmetic products:

- *Active ingredients*: how the active ingredients are sourced and processed is an important consideration for determining if the product should be considered organic.
- *Formulation:* for a product to be considered organic, it cannot contain synthetic chemicals.
- *Delivery system*: lab-produced delivery systems cannot generally be considered organic, although in the case of esthetic treatments removing layers of the stratum corneum is a tool used to enhance absorption into the skin.
- *Stability and safety*: it is important to remember that *natural* does not always mean safe. A preservative system must be used, and the product should be formulated in a way to guarantee stability.

The reality is that although active herbal ingredients do have active properties, those ingredients need to penetrate through the stratum corneum to impact the skin. This requires a delivery system, which cannot be considered organic when looking at the various certification guidelines.

Improving and maintaining the acid mantle is the best benefit organic skin care will have, unless there is a delivery system. This definitely does impact aging skin but works in a slower manner.

Guidelines

Only one United States agency exists that certifies organic foods, and that is the United States Department of Agriculture—the National Organic Program. All other guidelines with respect to organic foods are implemented by private associations. One example is **OASIS, Organic and Sustainable Industry Standards**, which is focused solely on health and beauty products; another is the National Products Association.

OASIS, Organic and Sustainable Industry Standards
international organization that certifies organic health and beauty products.

Unites States Department of Agriculture

In 1990 the United States Congress passed the Organic Foods Production Act (OFPA). This act required the USDA to develop standards for the production of organically produced agricultural products. The purpose of the OFPA is to:

1. To establish national standards governing the marketing of certain agricultural products that can be considered organically produced products.

2. To assure consumers that organically produced products meet a consistent standard.
3. To facilitate interstate commerce in fresh and processed food that is organically produced.

The National Organic Program administers the standards through the code of federal regulations, title 7, part 205, which enforces the Organic Foods Production Act. This standard is for agricultural products, not personal care products. If a personal care product contains or is made up of agricultural products and can meet the USDA Natural Organic Program standards, it may be eligible to be certified by a USDA accredited certifying agent.

After an agricultural product is certified, four organic label categories can be used based on their organic content:

- **100 percent organic:** the product must contain only organically produced ingredients excluding salt and water. The products can display USDA organic seal and must include the certifying agent's name and address. See Figure 12-3 for an example of the USDA organic seal.
- **Organic:** the product must contain 95 percent organically produced ingredients excluding water and salt. Remaining ingredients must consist of nonagricultural substances approved on the National List or nonorganically produced agricultural products that are not available in organic form.
- **Made with organic ingredients:** the product must contain at least 70 percent organic ingredients, and the product label can list up to three of the organic ingredients on the principal display panel. The product may *not* display the USDA organic seal.
- **Less than 70 percent organic ingredients:** products cannot use the term organic anywhere on the principal display panel. They can identify the specific ingredients that are USDA certified as organic. Products may *not* display the USDA organic seal.

In addition to the standards for labeling, there are production and handling standards. These standards address organic crop production, wild crop harvesting, livestock management, and processing of organic agricultural products.

Some of these standards are:

- Organic crops are grown without using conventional pesticides, petroleum-based fertilizers, or sewage sludge fertilizers.
- Genetic modification and ionizing radiation are prohibited, as are all synthetic substances unless listed on the National List of allowed synthetic substances.

A civil penalty of up to $11,000 can be levied on anyone misusing the USDA organic label.

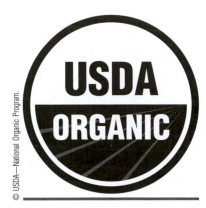

© USDA—National Organic Program.

Figure 12-3 USDA 100% organic seal indicates a product is 100% organic and must contain, excluding salt and water, only organically produced ingredients.

- Animals must be fed organic feed, given access to the outdoors, and given no antibiotics or growth hormones.

Ecocert

Ecocert is an international organization started in France in 1991. Ecocert primarily certifies food, in the same way as the USDA **National Organic Program (NOP)**, but has expanded into textiles, personal care products, detergents, and perfumes. Ecocert is utilized in 80 countries, and the international headquarters are in Germany. The goal of Ecocert is to:

1. Create standards of certification for organic products.
2. Set certification standards for fair trade.
3. Set certification of good agricultural processes (GAP) standards.

Ecocert has specific guidelines for organic cosmetics, and they offer two types of descriptions of organic products:

- **Natural and Organic:** 95 percent of plant ingredients are certified as organic, and the product contains 5 percent maximum synthetic ingredients. Products must have 10 percent of total ingredients certified as organic.
- **Natural:** 50 percent of plant ingredients are certified as organic. Products must have 5 percent of total ingredients certified as organic.

Ingredients not permitted are synthetic versions of the following:

- Emollients
- Perfumes
- Antioxidants
- Color
- Oils and fats
- Silicones

Also, ingredients and processes *not* allowed include the following:

- Ingredients created from petrochemicals
- Ingredients created from genetically modified organisms
- Any use of ionizing radiation
- Ingredients and finished products that generate the formation of nitrosamines
- Ingredients or products tested on animals

OASIS

Organic and Sustainable Industry Standards is an association that was started by a group of skin care product manufacturers who were

> More important than the organic certification is the issue of sustainability. Organic ingredients are good, but not at the cost of the environment. If the ingredient is a rare non-renewable source or a source that is slow to renew, the effects on the environment can be detrimental. The next issue is what the item is packaged in and how it is transported. As a lifestyle choice, classifying an item as *organic* requires much thought.

Ecocert
European organization; primarily certifies organic food but has expanded into textiles, personal care products, detergents, and perfumes.

National Organic Program (NOP)
American non-profit organization certifying natural food and personal products.

organic and sustainable industry standards

Figure 12–4 OASIS seal certifies standards for all aspects of personal care product manufacturing.

concerned about the *green washing* happening with the personal care industry. These standards cover all aspects of the personal care product manufacturing.

General Guidelines   The OASIS standard encompasses the verification of materials, processes, production, and conditions for health and beauty products to use organic label claims. OASIS standards are not to be used for certification for food products, only for products defined under state and federal regulations as cosmetics or other products that are sold in a health and beauty retail setting such as distributors of candles, soaps, and aromas. See Figure 12-4 for an example of the oasis seal.

OASIS standards do not verify product quality and raw materials and finished processed products must be certified to the USDA organic standards by an accredited USDA certifier.

Substances not allowed include the following:

- Ingredients produced at the farm level with sewage sludge
- Ingredients processed with ionizing radiation
- Ingredients that have been made with genetic engineering or from raw materials derived from plants grown with genetic engineering
- Ingredients with petroleum compounds, unless specifically allowed in the OASIS standard 100
- Formaldehyde or formaldehyde donors
- Substances produced from non-sustainable sources and with no organic substitutes
- Substances whose manufacture, use, and disposal have adverse effects on the environment and people

Product Production and Labeling Requirements   Three OASIS labels that can be used on products include:

- **100 Percent Organic:** any product sold with the 100 percent organic label must have by weight or volume (excluding salt and water) 100 percent certified organic ingredients. This includes any of the processing aids, catalysts, reagents, and other materials that may come into contact with the product. All processing aids must be plant derived.
- **Organic:** any product that uses the organic label must have by weight or volume (excluding salt and water) 90 percent organically produced raw or processed agricultural ingredients. Ten percent of the product must be organically produced unless it is not commercially available; ingredients can be nonagricultural or not organically produced if approved by OASIS standards.
- **Made with Organic:** products labeled made with organic must have by weight or volume (excluding salt and water) 70 percent

organically produced raw or processed agricultural ingredients. Soap is considered a *made with organic* product due to its chemical makeup. The remaining 30 percent of ingredients must be organically produced unless not commercially available; ingredients can be nonagricultural or not organically produced if approved.

Natural Products Association

Founded in 1936 as the American Health Foods Association, the National Products Association (NPA) is an American nonprofit organization certifying natural food and personal products. Their mission is to advocate for consumers as well as help create a broader, more accessible market for natural products. Their certification guidelines mimic the USDA's guidelines with the addition of the following:

- No ingredients that have a potential human health risk
- Ingredients must come from a renewable plentiful source in nature
- No processes can be used that would alter the effectiveness or purity of the natural ingredient

This organization creates an alternative to the consumer for quality control, which helps the natural products industry.

Green Chemistry or Sustainable Chemistry

Green chemistry is the use of processes that reduce the use or eliminate the generation of hazardous substances. This process governs the manufacture, handling, disposal, and processing of chemicals. The goals of green chemistry are:

- Reduced waste
- Safe products
- Reduced use of natural resources and energy

Green chemistry
the use of processes that reduce the use or eliminate the generation of hazardous substances.

The Environmental Protection Agency promotes the use of green chemistry through various programs and has based their guidelines on the 12 principles of green chemistry that were developed by Paul Anastas and John Warner in 1992.[1] They are:

- Prevent waste
- Atom economy, which is avoiding waste by incorporating the starting materials into the desired end product
- Use fewer hazardous chemicals
- Create safer chemicals
- Use safer solvents and other substances

- Observe energy efficiency
- Use renewable resources
- Reduce derivatives
- Use catalysis instead of **stoichiometric** reagents
- Design for degradation
- Prevent pollution
- Safer chemical use for accident prevention

stoichiometric
a reaction involving substances that are in exact proportions.

Green chemistry is important for estheticians to understand in order to educate their clients about the way their products are created as well as what the possible carbon footprint is for that product. Currently the federal government does not regulate green chemistry but the state of California does.

How to Decide to Go Green

The option of *going green* or using only organic products is only one part of creating a green or sustainable business. Going green requires looking at the whole picture, starting with where the ingredients are sourced and including how ingredients use energy to get to the business. Just because you have a natural ingredient as a source does not mean it is sustainable. There are many environmental impacts on sourcing rare or endangered ingredients for products. There may be benefits to the health of the person but negative effects on the environment. Some questions to ask before deciding on an organic skin care line are:

- How are the ingredients chosen?
  Ingredients should be chosen with efficacy, safety, and sustainability in mind.
- Are the ingredients USDA organic certified?
  For an agricultural product to be considered organic it must meet the USDA NOP requirements, unless an Ecocert qualification is being used.
- Where do the ingredients come from?
  If the ingredients are harvested from a distant location or are sourced far away from the manufacturing facility, this will increase the impact on the environment.
- Are the ingredients sustainable?
  Sustainable refers to plant sources that can be harvested annually, are not an endangered plant species, and whose harvest does not cause environmental damage.

- How are the ingredients prepared?
  Every plant extracted must be prepared in a lab before being used in a product. The extraction process and solvents used can negate the organic status of the product.
- Where are the products manufactured?
  A product manufactured and packaged from a distant place will add to the environmental damage due to the transportation of the product to the salon, spa, or clinic.
- How are the products packaged for transport and storage?
  Packaging is important for stability as well as recyclability. How the products are packaged for shipping is also important. Is the manufacturer a green manufacturer but using Styrofoam™ as packing material?
- Is the packaging recyclable and biodegradable?
  This is an important part of sustainability and green science. The packaging needs to be recyclable or the organic label is inefficient. Labels should utilize biodegradable ink and other materials considered green.
- What are the efficacy claims?
  Is the product line making substantial claims such as age reversal and use of organic products? If so, what proof is offered?
- What delivery systems do the products use?
  If a product is claiming specific results with the use of organically certified ingredients, what is the delivery system? If the product is using nanotechnology delivery systems or liposomes, can this be considered organic? Chapter 7 discusses information on delivery systems.

There are also ingredients that cause concern for clients and estheticians alike. The most common classes of ingredients causing concerns are parabens, phthalates, and sulfites. Refer to Chapter 7 for details on ingredients that cause concerns.

▶ ▷ ▷ Top Ten Tips to Take to the Clinic

1. Organic lifestyle is healthy to adopt and has many health benefits. It is hard to translate those standards to the personal care market, including professional-level products.

2. The term *organic* is truly used to describe a class of chemicals with a carbon basis, or living organism basis.

3. Unless there is a delivery system, the best benefit organic skin care can have is improving and maintaining the acid mantle, moisture content, and texture of the skin.

4. The United States Department of Agriculture National Organic Program is the only United States agency that certifies organic foods.

5. USDA guidelines for a label that states *100 percent organic* certify the product contains only organically produced ingredients, excluding salt and water.

6. The label *made with organic ingredients* from the USDA guidelines certifies the product contains at least 70 percent organic ingredients and a product label.

7. Ecocert guidelines for the label *Natural* are that 50 percent of plant ingredients are certified as organic. Products must have 5 percent of total ingredients certified as organic.

8. OASIS guidelines state that any products with a label of *organic* must have by weight or volume, excluding salt and water, 90 percent organically produced raw or processed agricultural ingredients.

9. Green chemistry is the use of processes that reduce the use or eliminate the generation of hazardous substances.

10. Sustainability and renewability is as important as how the ingredients are grown.

Chapter Review Questions

1. Can organic products impact aging skin?

2. What is the penalty for misusing the USDA organic label?

3. What four certifications can an organic product use if approved?

4. What is green chemistry?

5. Which state regulates green chemistry?

6. What questions should you ask yourself when considering an organic line?

References

1. Anastas, P. T., Warner, J. C. (1998). *Green Chemistry: Theory and Practice*. New York: Oxford University Press.

Bibliography

Baumann, L. MD., Saghari, S. MD., Weisburg, E. MS. (2009). *Cosmetic Dermatology: Principles and Practice*, 2nd Edition. New York: McGraw Hill Medical.

Websites

www.ams.usda.gov/nop
www.oasis.org
www.epa.gov/greenchemistry
www.ecocert.com
www.npainfo.org

Answers to Chapter Review Questions

Chapter 1

1. What is one of the definitions of *esthetician*?
   Answer: *A licensed professional who is an expert in the maintenance and improvement of healthy skin.*

2. Can an esthetician diagnose or treat any skin disease?
   Answer: *No, an esthetician cannot treat or diagnose any skin disease, or alter the structure and function of the skin without the supervision of a doctor.*

3. What are the areas of a client's life that need to be considered when approaching aging treatment holistically?
   Answer: *Lifestyle, personal stressors, medical history, skin care, attitude, and activity level.*

4. Can an esthetician offer advice to clients dealing with depression, anxiety, or grief issues?
   Answer: *No, refer them to a therapist or doctor.*

5. What are the signs of sensitive skin?
   Answer:
   - *Rough texture, resistant to treatment.*
   - *Redness in specific areas or widespread.*
   - *Inflammation, both chronic and acute.*
   - *Dryness, flakiness, and dehydration.*
   - *Feeling of stinging, burning, or general tightness; can happen without inflammation.*

Chapter 2

1. What are a few basic tips for encouraging positive communication?
   Answer: *Tips for mastering good communication include listening, asking open-ended questions, maintaining eye contact and positive body language, and not interrupting during the conversation. It is best to keep the focus on the client, and keep communication clear by avoiding industry terms or slang that a client may not be familiar with.*

2. List ways in which you can portray professionalism and ethics as a skin care professional.
   Answer: *Estheticians should maintain client confidentiality, keep treatment and documentation records, and provide clear, honest communication. Be sure to provide clients with clear and realistic goals and outcomes, and adhere to the scope of practice of the profession. Refer clients to the appropriate qualified health practitioner when indicated. You can also stay up-to-date by seeking out continuing education, and dress in attire consistent with professional practice.*

3. Explain ways to accommodate and work with physically challenged clients in the treatment room.
    Answer:
    - *Use an electric or hydraulic treatment table.*
    - *Help your client on and off the treatment table.*
    - *Use a heated pad and heated mitts during treatment, as heat can naturally lessen the pain if your client is not intolerant to it.*
    - *Use a back, neck, and shoulder support, depending on the client's level of disability. Lying completely flat can cause additional pain.*
    - *Keep at-home care simple. Many clients with arthritis have problems with spreading products on the skin and opening jars. Pumps, sprays, and large wide jars are easier for clients with severe arthritis to handle. Makeup brush handles should be longer and have a larger handle.*
    - *Always communicate with your clients about how they feel.*
    - *Keep artificial fragrance to a minimum.*
    - *Use clear written instructions for clients' home care and treatment descriptions.*
    - *Keep clutter to a minimum.*

4. What are some of the guidelines for handling emotions in the treatment room?
    Answer:
    - *Stay calm.*
    - *Do not try to solve the client's problem.*
    - *Use good listening skills and offer support when appropriate.*
    - *Do not give advice; stay neutral. For example, say, "I am sorry you are feeling so down, angry, sad, disappointed." If the environment is subdued, calm, and relaxing, often all that is needed are simple environmental cues, such as music, tea, water, soothing and comforting items.*

    - *Do not try to be a therapist; in fact, you might have a supply of information on local therapists whom clients could consult.*
    - *Limit the conversation. It's best to say little, give an excellent massage, and direct clients in breathing and relaxing while you give them their treatment.*

5. What are some tips for marketing to the healthy aging client?
    Answer:
    - *Educate your client.*
    - *Listen. Clients need to feel that their needs are being met.*
    - *Understand. Recognize client challenges and offer solutions. This is the key to offering results-oriented treatments.*
    - *Create a service brand. This principle starts with respect, which turns to loyalty that leads to a positive professional—client relationship. Respect from the customer towards you as a professional and from the professional to the client is important.*

Chapter 3

1. What should you do if a liability situation occurs during a treatment?
    Answer:
    - *Have products available specifically for soothing the skin such as colloidal oatmeal, aloe vera, hydrocortisone, gel masks, or whatever your manufacturer recommends.*
    - *Contact the manufacturer immediately via phone.*
    - *Document phone call and instructions given.*

2. What are the characteristics of dry skin?
    Answer:
    - *Pores are fine, almost invisible.*
    - *Texture is smooth and fine.*
    - *Under a Woods lamp skin will show a white fluorescence.*

3. What are the characteristics of oily skin?
   Answer:
   - *Pore size is large and visible throughout the face.*
   - *Texture can feel like an orange peel (rough and thick).*
   - *Tone will have a shine with obvious oil.*
   - *There are no areas of dryness but the skin can be dehydrated.*
   - *Under a Woods lamp you will see small orange dots throughout the face.*

4. What are the characteristics of combination skin?
   Answer:
   - *Pore size can range from small to large, but pores are located only through the center panel of the face; the typical T-zone.*
   - *Texture can be rough in some areas and smooth in others.*
   - *There will be conditions associated with this skin type.*
   - *Under a Woods lamp the skin will show small orange dots where sebum is being produced.*

5. What questions should you ask your client to determine a client's healing response time?
   Answer:
   - *Do you bruise easily?*
   - *How long does it take to heal from a cut?*
   - *Do discolorations form after the cut heals?*
   - *Do discolorations form after having a blemish?*
   - *Have you had melasma from pregnancy?*
   - *Do you scar easily?*
   - *Is it keloid scarring or atrophic scarring?*
   - *Have you had aesthetic medical treatments such as lasers, IPL, radiofrequency, or plastic surgery?*
   - *How did your skin react after the treatment?*

Chapter 4

1. What are the most widely accepted aging theories?
   Answer:
   - *Free radical theory*
   - *Membrane theory*
   - *Neuroendocrine theory*
   - *Inflammation theory*
   - *Cross linking theory*
   - *Telomerase theory*
   - *Mitochondrial theory*

2. What is the term *senescence* related to?
   Answer: *The term* senescence *is used to refer to the biological process of aging and is used to define an entire body of scientific study.*

3. What is macro aging?
   Answer: *Macro aging refers to the signs of aging that are visible.*

4. What is micro aging?
   Answer: *Micro aging refers to the aging that is happening at the cellular level.*

5. What is the telomerase theory of aging?
   Answer: *Telomeres shorten each time a cell divides, which leads to cellular damage due to the cell not being able to duplicate itself correctly. Each time this damaged cell duplicates itself it becomes worse and eventually dies. This leads to cellular dysfunction, aging, and death.*

6. What is the inflammation theory of aging?
   Answer: *The inflammation theory of aging states that the long-term effects of chronic inflammation result in accumulated damage to the body.*

Chapter 5

1. What is the function of the acid mantle?
   Answer: *Maintains skin pH, inhibits growth of harmful bacteria, and prevents TEWL.*

2. What is the function of the stratum granulosum?

Answer: *The stratum granulosum is responsible for the formation of amino acids that create natural moisture factor (NMF) and dissolving of the desmosomes.*

3. What is the function of the stratum basale?

Answer: *The stratum basale is responsible for maintaining the epidermis by continually renewing, RETE pegs connect the epidermis to dermis, melanocytes are found here, TA cells are responsible for the most cell division.*

4. What are the diagnostic signs of stage 1 aging skin?

Answer:
- *Fine texture changes—general roughness*
- *Fine lines visible with facial movement*
- *Dynamic expression lines*
- *Mild hyperpigmentation or general dull appearance to skin*
- *Nasolabial fold beginning to become pronounced*
- *Mild skin fold at edge of ear when lying down*
- *Photodamage apparent under Woods lamp*
- *Increased dryness or dehydration*
- *Increased redness or sensitivity*
- *Small vertical lines found at tear ducts and lash line and rough texture around eyes*
- *Small vertical lines on upper lip area*

5. What are the subtypes of rosacea?

Answer:
- *Subtype 1: Erythematotelangiectatic Rosacea*
- *Subtype 2: Papulopustular Rosacea*
- *Subtype 3: Phymatous Rosacea*
- *Subtype 4: Ocular Rosacea*

Chapter 6

1. What is the purpose of the cleansing phase?

Answer: *The purpose of the cleansing phase is the removal of debris from stratum corneum for a clear analysis of skin, and to prepare the skin for a second cleansing.*

2. What is the purpose of the exfoliation phase?

Answer: *The exfoliation phase removes the stratum corneum in a controlled manner to activate the skin's wound healing response.*

3. What is the purpose of the active infusion phase?

Answer: *The active infusion phase introduces specific ingredients into the epidermis that will influence specific cellular reactions within the skin.*

4. What benefits does massage provide the skin?

Answer: *Benefits include increases in micro-circulation to bring oxygen and nutrients to cells; induces the relaxation response; improves lymph circulation for removal of toxins as well as increasing epidermal hydration (free water content); stimulates cellular function, aids in desquamation; stimulates sebaceous glands; and facilitates penetration of active ingredients.*

5. What types of exfoliation are good for hyperpigmentation?

Answer: *Lactic acid, glycolic, Jessner's, and proteolytic enzymes.*

Chapter 7

1. What is the FDA definition of cosmetics?

Answer: *The definition of cosmetics is "articles intended to be rubbed, poured, sprinkled, or sprayed on, introduced into, or otherwise applied to the human body or any part thereof for cleansing, beautifying, promoting attractiveness, or altering the appearance and articles intended for use as a component of any such articles; except that such term shall not include soap."*

2. How far does UVA penetrate skin?

Answer: *UVA can penetrate the dermis.*

3. Does SPF rating indicate protection against all UV radiation?
Answer: *No, the SPF rating indicates protection only against UVB.*

4. What is the difference between a chemical and physical sunscreen ingredient?
Answer: *Physical sunscreen ingredients reflect UVR; chemical ingredients absorb it.*

5. Have parabens been proven to be toxic?
Answer: *No, it is still a theory.*

Chapter 8

1. What does LASER stand for?
Answer: *Laser stands for light amplification by the stimulated emission of radiation.*

2. What are ANSI standards?
Answer: *ANSI or American National Standards Institute standards regulate the safe use of lasers in healthcare facilities.*

3. How long should you wait before doing a facial treatment on a client who has had a Botox injection?
Answer: *A client should wait 48–72 hours before receiving a facial after having Botox injections.*

4. What is cell therapy and what is the proposed benefit of this treatment?
Answer: *Cell therapy is a new type of non-invasive anti-aging treatment that extracts fibroblasts from the patient's skin, causes them to multiply into millions of new cells, freezes them, and then reinjects the cells back into the patient's skin. It is proposed to increase the skin's ability to create collagen.*

5. What is the esthetician's role in aesthetic medical treatments?
Answer: *The esthetician's role in aesthetic medical treatments is to support and educate the client, and get their skin into healthy shape.*

Chapter 9

1. Describe stress.
Answer: *Stress is a physical and mental response to stressors.*

2. What are some of the causes of stress?
Answer: *Causes of stress can be death of a loved one, financial problems, relationship problems, or chronic pain.*

3. What is the right amount of sleep?
Answer: *The right amount of sleep, is seven to nine hours.*

4. List coping strategies to help manage stress.
Answer: *Coping strategies can be massage, meditation, healthy sleep, and fitness.*

5. What are the signs of smoking in the skin?
Answer:
- *Increased wrinkling*
- *Red and orange complexion*
- *Ashy pale coloring*
- *Puffiness*
- *Gauntness and loss of elasticity*
- *Yellow, irregularly thickened skin*
- *Increased pre-cancerous lesions*

Chapter 10

1. What are the best supplement recommendations for aging skin?
Answer: **Vitamins** *(Vitamin A, Biotin, Niacin, D_3);* **Antioxidants** *(Vitamin C, Vitamin E, Coenzyme Q10, Lycopene, Green Tea, Silymarin, Resveratrol, Grape Seed Extract, Pomegranate Extract, Pycnogenol, Omega-3, Omega-6 Fatty Acids);* **Minerals** *(Zinc, Hyaluronic Acid, Glucosamine, DHEA).*

2. What is the recommended water intake?
Answer: *The recommended water intake is 0.5 ounces per pound of body weight.*

3. What foods and drinks should clients with rosacea skin avoid?

Answer: *Clients with rosacea should avoid hot spicy food and alcohol.*

4. What foods should skin prone to acne avoid?
Answer: *Clients prone to acne should avoid iodine and milk.*

5. What do dietary recommendations always start with?
Answer: *Dietary recommendations always start with a healthy aging consultation.*

Chapter 11

1. What benefits does exercise provide skin?
Answer: *Exercise increases circulation for both the lymphatic as well as vascular system and helps to reduce stress.*

2. How many days per week should strength training be done?
Answer: *Strength training can occur three to four days with at least 24–48 hours recovery time between sessions.*

3. What is the recommended plan for beginner physical fitness described by the government?
Answer: *The recommendation for beginners is 150 minutes (2 hours and 30 minutes) of moderate intensity aerobic activity or 75 minutes (1 hour and 15 min) of vigorous intensity aerobic activity. It is best performed in at least 10-minute increments weekly and can also be combined intensities.*

4. How many days per week can yoga be done?
Answer: *Yoga can be performed daily.*

5. What is hGH?
Answer: *hGH is a hormone secreted by the anterior pituitary gland in pulses throughout the day; it declines as we age.*

6. Why is hGH important to skin?
Answer: *hGH is involved with most physiological processes within the body and has an impact on fat metabolism, muscle mass, bone density, collagen formation, and maintenance.*

7. Why is chronic stress bad for the body?
Answer: *Chronic stress leads to subclinical inflammation, which is also implicated in premature aging and disease.*

Chapter 12

1. Can organic products impact aging skin?
Answer: *Yes, organic products can benefit mature skin if they are formulated to improve the acid mantle and stratum corneum of the skin.*

2. What is the penalty for misusing the USDA Organic label?
Answer: *An $11,000 fine is the penalty for misusing the USDA Organic label.*

3. What four certifications can an organic product use if approved?
Answer: *USDA, Ecocert, OASIS, and Natural Products Association are the four approved certifications.*

4. What is green chemistry?
Answer: *Green chemistry is the use of processes that reduce the use or eliminate the generation of hazardous substances.*

5. Which state regulates green chemistry?
Answer: *The state of California regulates green chemistry.*

6. What questions should you ask yourself when considering an organic line?
Answer:
- *How are the ingredients chosen?*
- *Are the ingredients USDA Organic certified?*
- *Where do the ingredients come from?*
- *Are the ingredients sustainable?*
- *How are the ingredients prepared?*
- *Where are the products manufactured?*
- *How are the products packaged?*
- *Is the packaging recyclable and biodegradable?*
- *What are the efficacy claims?*
- *What delivery systems do the products use?*

Glossary

7-dehydrocholestrol fatty acid fatty acid that provides the body with vitamin d3 through the conversion of ultraviolet light.

A

acid (dehydrocholesterol fatty) a fatty acid involved in the skin's process of converting UV radiation to vitamin D.

acid mantle skin layer that is a complex fluid at a pH of 4.5 to 5.5 formed by the excretions from sebaceous, sudoriferous glands, epidermal lipids, and NMF (natural moisture factor); contains 7-dehydrocholesterol fatty acid. This layer has *micro flora* that contribute to the skin's first layer barrier defense.

adenosine triphosphate (ATP) this molecule provides cellular energy transport and enzyme regulation.

adrenocorticotropic hormone (ACTH) hormone secreted by the pituitary in response to stress.

advanced glycation end products (AGEs) process of glycation; binds a sugar molecule to protein, which creates oxidative stress and increases inflammatory cytokines.

alipidic oil dry skin.

American National Standards Institute (ANSI) standards for the safe use of lasers in healthcare facilities.

anaphylactic rapidly developing and serious allergic reaction that affects a number of different areas of the body at one time.

anion when electrolytes are dissolved in water, they split and form ions that carry either a positive or negative charge. A negatively charged ion is an anion.

anode when galvanic current is introduced into the electrolyte solution, the ions move to either the positive pole, called the anode, or the negative pole, called the cathode.

AP-1 transcription factor which regulates gene expression and controls cellular processes in response to a variety of stimuli, including cytokines, growth factors, stress, and bacterial and viral infections.

aquaporin channels water channels that transport water across cell membranes made of specialized membrane proteins known as aquaporins. Discovered by Peter Agre, who jointly won a Nobel Prize in 2003.

atrophic crinkling rhytids fine horizontal and parallel wrinkles that tend to form later in life; they can occur anywhere on the face and body.

C

calcitonin gene-related peptide (CGRP) regulates the antigen presenting function of the Langerhans cells.

cathode when galvanic current is introduced into the electrolyte solution, the ions move to either the positive pole, called the anode, or the negative pole, called the cathode.

cation when electrolytes are dissolved in water, they split and form ions that carry either a positive or negative charge. A positively charged ion is a cation.

cavitation formation and collapse of bubbles in a liquid by means of a mechanical force.

ceramide a molecule within the lipid family, made of a sphingosine plus a fatty acid, naturally found within the skin.

cholesterol thick lipid molecule found within cell membranes and transported within blood plasma; needed for healthy cell function.

chromosomes organized structure of DNA and protein found within cells.

chronic obstructive pulmonary disease (COPD) a progressive disease that makes it hard to breathe.

collagenase an enzyme that controls the removal of collagen within the body.

comedones sebaceous secretions that become trapped with skin pores. They can appear as open comedones (blackheads) or closed comedomes (whiteheads).

corneocytes cells without a nucleus and cellular structure; they are filled with keratin proteins, with lipids surrounding them in the extracellular space.

corynebacterium gram-positive rod-shaped bacteria; can be harmful to humans.

cosmeceuticals a term coined by Dr. Albert Kligman to describe topical cosmetics that are designed to improve the appearance of the skin through delivery of active ingredients into the epidermis.

cosmetic sensitivity skin that cannot tolerate certain cosmetics, usually fragrances, and preservatives.

D

desmosomes small hair-like protrusions that hold cells together; integral for cell transport.

desquamation turnover of dead cells. Shedding or peeling of the outermost layer of skin.

diffuse redness also known as *erythema*, general redness in the skin. This can indicate a sensitive skin.

dopamine receptors receptors found in the central nervous sytem and key organs that help regulate dopamine, which is essential for proper nerve function. A disruption in dopamine results in mood disorders, poor memory, and cognitive dysfunction.

dynamic expression lines aging lines that are more apparent with facial movement.

dyschromia disorder of pigmentation in skin and hair.

E

Ecocert European organization; primarily certifies organic food but has expanded into textiles, personal care products, detergents, and perfumes.

edema extracellular water that becomes trapped and causes swelling.

elastase the enzyme that activates elastosis.

elastosis loss of elasticity; the breakdown of elastin fibers within the skin.

electrolytes ionized solutions are called electrolytes; they are conductors of electricity.

eleidin precursor molecule to the formation of keratin.

environmental sensitivity irritated easily by sun and wind exposure.

epidermal growth factor (EGF) a protein molecule or steroid hormone that stimulates proliferation and differentiation of epidermal cells.

epidermal growth factor receptor (EGFR) a receptor found in epidermal cells that enables EGF to function.

epidermal lipids important part of the structure of the epidermis; prevents TEWL. Includes triglycerides, fatty acids, squalene, wax esters, and cholesterol; can be affected by diet, genetics, environment, and aging.

ER-A androgen receptor and estrogen receptor found on skin cells.

ER-B an estrogen receptor found on skin cells. Second type found.

erythema also known as *diffuse redness*; increased circulation within the skin that manifests as redness.

essential fatty acid fatty acids found to be essential for proper cellular functions. These are often identified as omega acids 3 and 6, found in fatty fish and some nuts and oils.

essential fatty acid deficiency (EFAD) lack of essential fatty acids such as omegas 3 and 6. The body cannot manufacture essential fatty acids as they must be ingested.

esthetician (or aesthetician) a licensed professional who is an expert on maintaining and improving healthy skin.

excoriations a condition in which patients produce skin lesions, scratches, and irritation through repetitive, compulsive picking of their skin.

extracellular matrix (ECM) a network of non-living tissues that provides support, regulates communication, and encourages growth, healing, and adhesion for cells. Skin has a large extracellular matrix that keeps the skin strong and young looking.

extraction technique used to remove comedones, milia, and pustules from skin. Tools and manual pressure may be used.

extrinsic aging visible signs of aging caused by external lifestyle factors.

F

fascia a sheet or band of fibrous connective tissue enveloping, separating, or binding together muscles, organs, and other soft structures of the body.

fibrillin small fibers that are a component of elastin.

fibroblasts cells in connective tissue that synthesize collagen.

fibrocyte long spindle-shaped cells found along bundles of collagen that are the principle cells of connective tissue; they help maintain the ground substance of the dermis.

fibromyalgia a condition that is defined by widespread muscle pain, fatigue, headaches, sleep disturbance, physiological stress, and problems with thinking.

fibronection a cell adhesion molecule that anchors cells to collagen or proteoglycans.

filaggrin filament aggregating protein; binds keratin filaments to form a structural matrix in the stratum corneum; the breakdown of filaggrin contributes to NMF (natural moisturizing factor).

Fitzpatrick typing a skin typing program based on the client's melanin production within the skin. This program can determine a client's ability to heal after aggressive treatments such as chemical peels and lasers.

folliculitis ingrown hair.

fractionated laser utilizes the 1550 nm wavelength and targets water in the skin, which leaves the stratum corneum attached.

free radical an atom or group of atoms that has at least one unpaired electron and is therefore unstable and highly reactive. Free radicals can damage cells and are believed to accelerate the progression of cancer, cardiovascular disease, and age-related diseases.

free sterols group of natural steroid alcohols, such as cholesterol and ergosterol, which are waxy insoluble substances.

G

gerontology the scientific study of the biological, psychological, and sociological phenomena associated with old age and aging.

Glogau Photodamage Classification Scale developed by Richard G. Glogau, MD, a clinical professor of dermatology at the University of California, San Francisco. It was created in order to objectively measure the severity of photoaging.

glycoproteins any of a group of conjugated proteins having a carbohydrate as the nonprotein component; important membrane proteins, which play a role in cell-to-cell interactions.

glycosaminoglycans GAGs form an important component of connective tissues.

gravitational fold deep wrinkle; this is a deep groove that is long and straight and can occur anywhere on the face.

green chemistry the use of processes that reduce the use or eliminate the generation of hazardous substances.

ground state state of least possible energy or zero energy point.

H

Health Insurance Portability and Accountability Act (HIPAA) legislation that protects the privacy of individually identifiable health information; includes the HIPAA Security Rule, which sets national standards for the security of electronic protected health information; and the confidentiality provisions of the Patient Safety Rule, which protect identifiable information being used to analyze patient safety events and improve patient safety.

holistic esthetics looking at the lifestyle, nutrition, physical fitness and daily care when treating their skin.

human growth hormone (hGH) hGH is a hormone involved with most physiological processes within the body and has an impact on fat metabolism, muscle mass, bone density, and collagen formation and maintenance.

humectant a class of cosmetic ingredients that attract water with in the skin.

hydrophilic attracted to water molecules.

hyperhydrosis over-hydrated skin.

hyperkeratosis increased build up of dead skin cells.

hyperpigmentation overproduction of melanin resulting from ultraviolet radiation or injury.

I

inert will not react with other ingredients.

inflammatory cytokines any of a number of small proteins that are secreted by specific cells of the immune system which carry signals locally between cells, to increase inflammation in response to immune system activation.

International Nomenclature of Cosmetic Ingredients (INCI) a system of names for cosmetic ingredients used internationally by chemists and regulators.

interpersonal skills ability to interact with clients.

interstitial fluid water found between the cells of the body that provides much of the liquid environment of the body.

intrinsic aging aging that is influenced by genetics.

ionized solution ionized solutions are called electrolytes; they are conductors of electricity.

iontophoresis ionized solutions are used under the electrodes to facilitate absorption into the epidermis, a process known as iontophoresis.

K

keloid raised scarring that forms beyond the borders of the original injury; caused by an overgrowth of granulation tissue, collagen type 3.

keratin (keratinized) skin cells with no nucleus found in the stratum corneum.

keratinization process in which desmosomes are not dissolving efficiently, which causes a dead skin cell buildup.

keratinocyte growth factor (KGF) a growth factor present in the epithelialization-phase of wound healing. In this phase, keratinocytes are covering the wound, forming the epithelium.

keratohyalin granules any of the irregularly shaped granules present in the cells of the granular layer of the epidermis.

keratosis pilaris genetic follicular condition that appears as red raised bumps on the skin.

krill common name given to shrimp-like marine crustaceans.

L

lacunae see *sonophoresis*.

lamellar bodies formed in the keratinocytes of the stratum spinosum and stratum granulosum. When the keratinocyte matures to the stratum corneum, enzymes degrade the outer envelope of the lamellar bodies, releasing types of lipids called free fatty acids and ceramides.

lamin fibrous proteins providing structural function and communication regulation within the cell.

Langerhans cells important part of the immune system found in skin; digests antigens.

laser acronym for *light amplification by the stimulated emission of radiation;* laser technology emits photons in a coherent beam. A laser has three parts: *energy source, active medium,* and *optical cavity.*

M

macro aging refers to the signs of aging that are visible.

manual lymphatic drainage (MLD) massage technique used to move lymph fluid to lymph nodes.

mast cells play a central role in inflammatory and immediate allergic reactions, found in tissues throughout the body, particularly in association with structures such as blood vessels and nerves.

melanin-stimulating hormone (MSH) responsible for starting the process of pigment creation.

melanocortin a cellular receptor on the melanocyte which melanin-stimulating hormone adheres to.

melanocytes melanin-producing cells located in the stratum basale.

melanosome the organelle of the melanocyte that is the pigment carrier.

melasma pregnancy mask.

metabolic syndrome three or more disorders related to your metabolism at the same time, which includes obesity (particularly around the waist area having an apple shape), a systolic (top number) blood pressure measurement higher than 120 or a diastolic (bottom number) blood pressure measurement higher than 80, elevated level of triglycerides and low low-density lipoprotein, resistance to insulin.

micro aging refers to the aging that is happening at the cellular level.

microorganisms microscopic forms of life such as gram-positive and -negative bacteria, yeast, and fungus.

mid-life astonishment theory that defines what happens to women in late mid-life, usually 50s and 60s. This is characterized by an amazement and despair of losing one's physical and sexual attractiveness, multiple losses accompanied by age, awareness of accelerated aging both physically and mentally as well as culture's stigmatization of aging.

milia term for whiteheads.

N

national organic program (NOP) American non-profit organization certifying natural food and personal products.

natural moisture factor (NMF) released by lamellar bodies, by-products of the breakdown of filaggrin; composed of amino acids; allows the stratum corneum to absorb water; important for enzymes to function; declines with age; dysfunction of this system is theorized to contribute to chronic inflammation thus aging.

negative pole creates an alkaline reaction that is vasodilative; this increases microcirculation, stimulates nerve tissues, causes saponification, and softens tissues.

NICE concept concept which states that the nervous, immune, cutaneous, and endocrine systems all work together to activate healthy skin function by the secretion of homeostasin.

nonsteroidal anti-inflammatory drug (NSAID) medications used primarily to treat inflammation, mild to moderate pain, and fever.

nucleic acids any of a group of complex compounds found in all living cells and viruses, composed of purines, pyrimidines, carbohydrates, and phosphoric acid. Nucleic acids in the form of DNA and RNA control cellular function and heredity.

O

odland bodies secretory organelles found in stratum granulosum layer of the epidermis; lamellar bodies are released from keratinocytes into the intercellular spaces to form an impermeable, lipid-containing sheet that serves to form a water barrier.

organic used to describe a class of chemicals with a carbon basis, or living organism.

Organic and Sustainable Industry Standards (OASIS) international organization that certifies organic health and beauty products.

osmotic pressure hydrostatic pressure caused by a difference in the amounts of solutes between solutions that are separated by a semipermeable membrane.

P

permanent elastotic creases wrinkles that are present without facial movement.

phagocytes white blood cells that protect the body by ingesting (phagocytosing) harmful foreign particles, bacteria, and dead or dying cells.

phospholipids lipids that are part of the cell membrane.

piezoelectric effect electrical charge created when the crystal is subjected to mechanical pressure.

pigmented lesions melanin in the skin.

Pilates form of exercise created by Joseph Pilates which focuses on core strength.

polypeptide growth factors protein that controls proliferation, cellular differentiation, and other functions in most cells.

POMC (proopiomelanocortin) secreted by the pituitary gland to activate melanin-stimulating hormone

positive pole when galvanic current is introduced into the electrolyte solution, the ions begin to move to either the positive pole, called the anode, or the negative pole, called the cathode.

professionalism the characteristics of a member of a vocation that has specialized vocational training.

profilaggrin a structural protein synthesized by cells of the stratum granulosum and a precursor of filaggrin.

Propionibacterium (P. Acnes) this bacteria helps with the creation of free fatty acids that are responsible for the acid pH of the acid mantle; it is also a factor in acne.

proteasome enzyme complex a protein group found within the cells; degrades and digests damaged proteins through proteolysis.

proteoglycans a glycoprotein that is a major component of the extracellular matrix

R

rate of perceived exertion (RPE) a system of determining workout intensity based on how the client feels during exercise and rates the intensity on a scale of 1–10.

reactive oxygen species (ROS) term used to describe free radicals due to the fact that most significant free radicals are oxygen centered.

RETE ridges epidermal thickenings that extend downward between dermal papillae.

rhytids wrinkles.

rosacea chronic skin condition involving inflammation of nose, cheeks, chin, and forehead.

Rubin classification of aging aging skin analysis developed by Dr. Mark Rubin.

S

saponification chemical processes that produce soap from fatty acid derivatives.

scarred ostia scarred follicles.

sebaceous hyperplasia a disorder of the sebaceous glands in which they become enlarged, causing clogged pores and raised milia-like bumps.

sebaceous secretions Sebum produced from the sebaceous gland.

seborrhea an inflammatory skin disorder affecting the scalp, face, and trunk, causing scaly, flaky, itchy, red skin.

self-objectification the tendency for women to evaluate themselves based on their physical appearance because they believe that this is how others judge them.

senescence process of cell aging.

SOAP (Subjective, Objective, Assessment and Plan) a charting system used in the medical community to identify issues the client feels (subjective) issues that the professional sees (objective) and then provide and accurate assessment or diagnosis to implement a plan for treatment.

solar lentigines freckles.

somatic cells one of the cells that take part in the formation of the body.

sonophoresis action caused by low-level ultrasound that is used to penetrate active ingredients through channels called lacunae.

sphingolipids lipids derived from sphingosine; important for cell functions.

Staphylococcus aureus gram-positive bacteria that is the most common cause of staph infections.

Staphylococcus epidermidis gram-positive bacteria that is part of the skin's natural micro flora.

static rhytids wrinkles that do not move with facial expression.

stoichiometric a reaction involving substances that are in exact proportions.

stress term commonly used to describe a physical and mental response to stressors.

Swami Sivananda Rahda yoga guru who modified the five principles of yoga for Western culture.

systemic sensitivity Sensitive to environmental insults; internal sensitivity; can be made worse by allergies, medication, and disease; sensitivity caused by internal factors.

T

TA (transient amplifying) cells cells that are involved in differentiation; also called daughter cells.

tactile sensitivity client feels uncomfortable when certain fabrics or pressures are used on the skin. Even towels can feel uncomfortable.

Tai Chi also referred to as *Tai Chi Chuan*; an ancient martial arts form that is used as a gentle meditative exercise.

Tai Chi Chuan see Tai Chi.

Tan Tien chi energy stored in the lower abdomen.

telangiectasia couperose, or broken capillaries.

telomerase an enzyme that adds DNA sequence.

telomeres region of repetitive DNA at the end of a chromosome, which protects the end of the chromosome from deterioration.

TGF-a protein that controls proliferation, cellular differentiation, and other functions in most cells.

TGF-b protein that controls proliferation, cellular differentiation, and other functions in most cells.

transepidermal water loss (TEWL) the process that allows epidermal water loss; impacted by an impaired acid mantle.

transglutaminases (TGase) involved in the formation of the cornified cell envelope by cross linking a variety of structural proteins in the epidermis.

tyrosinase enzyme that synthesizes tyrosine and L-dopa to create the melanosome.

tyrosine kinase activity a group of enzymes important in cell growth, differentiation, and development.

V

vascular lesions ruptures or malformations of blood vessels near the skin's surface. Common types include broken capillaries, spider veins, port wine stains, and hemangiomas.

vasoconstrictive constriction of blood vessels.

vasodilative relaxing or enlarging of blood vessels.

vesicles small sacs containing fluid.

Y

Yoga an ancient system of spiritual practice that includes body strengthening, which started as early as 3000 B.C.

Z

zazen one of the most common types of meditation.

Index

Note: page numbers followed by f or t refer to Figures or Tables